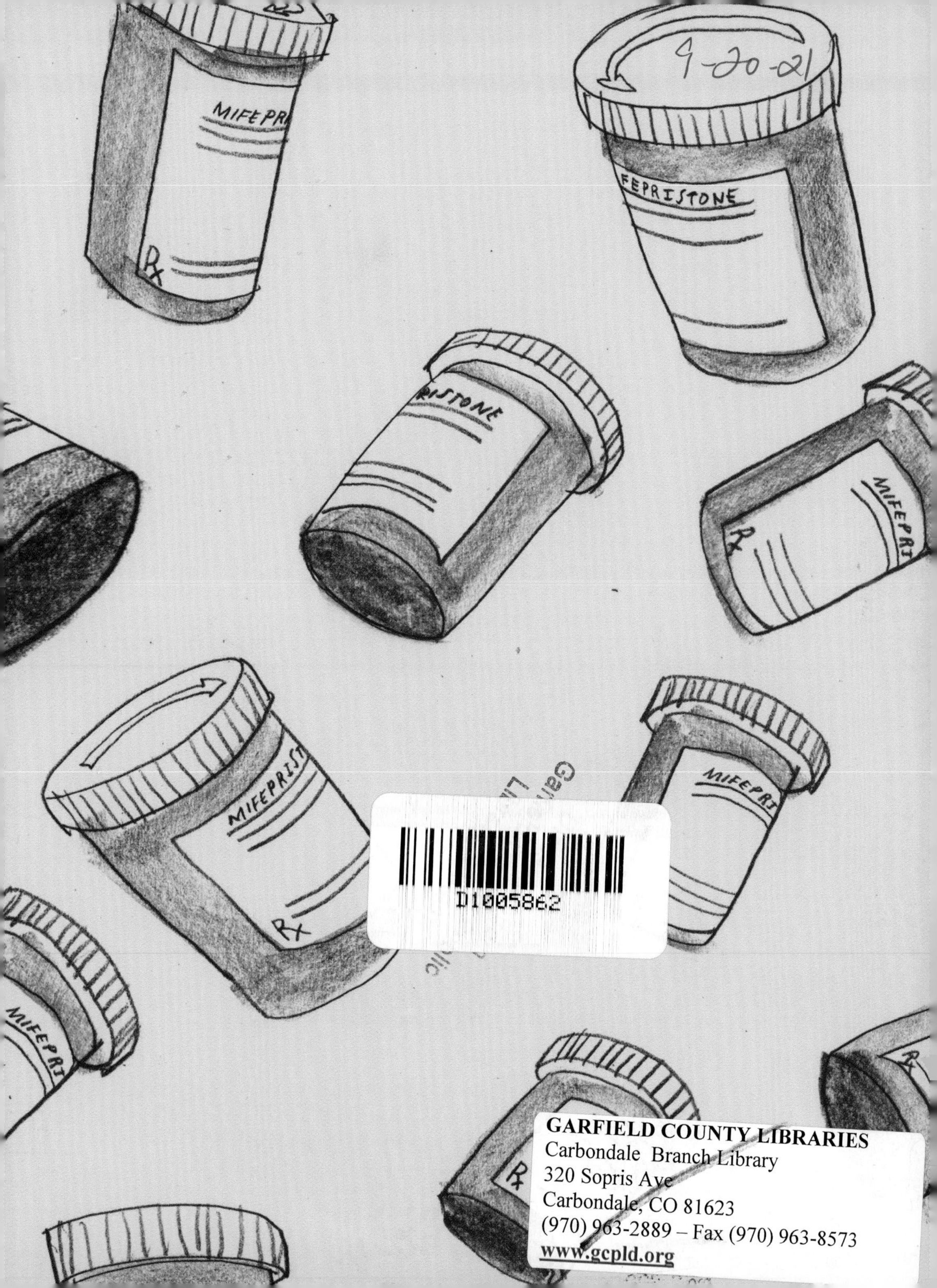
MIFEPRI
Rx
FEPRISTONE
RISTONE
MIFEPRI
Rx
MIFEPRIST
Rx
MIFEPRI
MIFEPRI
Rx
Rx

NOT FUNNY HA-HA

"NOT FUNNY HA-HA" BY LEAH HAYES
FANTAGRAPHICS BOOKS, 2015

EDITOR AND ASSOCIATE PUBLISHER: ERIC REYNOLDS
BOOK DESIGN: KEELI McCARTHY
PRODUCTION: PAUL BARESH
PUBLISHER: GARY GROTH

FANTAGRAPHICS BOOKS, INC.
SEATTLE WASHINGTON. USA
"NOT FUNNY HA-HA" IS COPYRIGHT © 2015 LEAH HAYES.

THIS EDITION IS COPYRIGHT © 2015 FANTAGRAPHICS
BOOKS, INC.

PERMISSION TO REPRODUCE CONTENT MUST BE
OBTAINED FROM THE AUTHOR OR PUBLISHER
ISBN 978-1-60699-839-7
LIBRARY OF CONGRESS CONTROL NUMBER: 2014960289
FIRST PRINTING: JUNE 2015
PRINTED IN MALAYSIA

A HANDBOOK FOR SOMETHING
HARD.

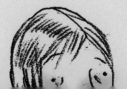

THIS BOOK IS FOR ALL
GIRLS AND WOMEN, AND
FOR THE PARTNERS, FRIENDS,
AND FAMILY WHO LOVE THEM.

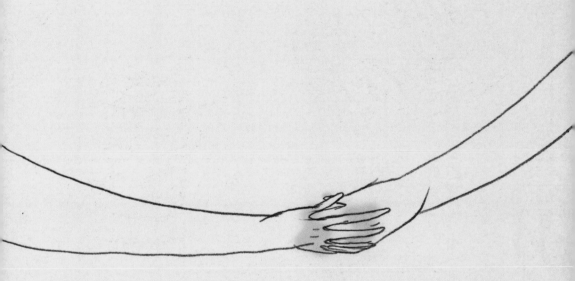

THANK YOU TO MY INCREDIBLE
FAMILY WHO HAS BEEN THERE
FOR ME THROUGH ALL OF THE
GOOD, BAD, AND FUNNY TIMES.

AND TO MY BUBBA... WHO STARTED A
LONG LINE OF AUDACIOUS WOMEN.

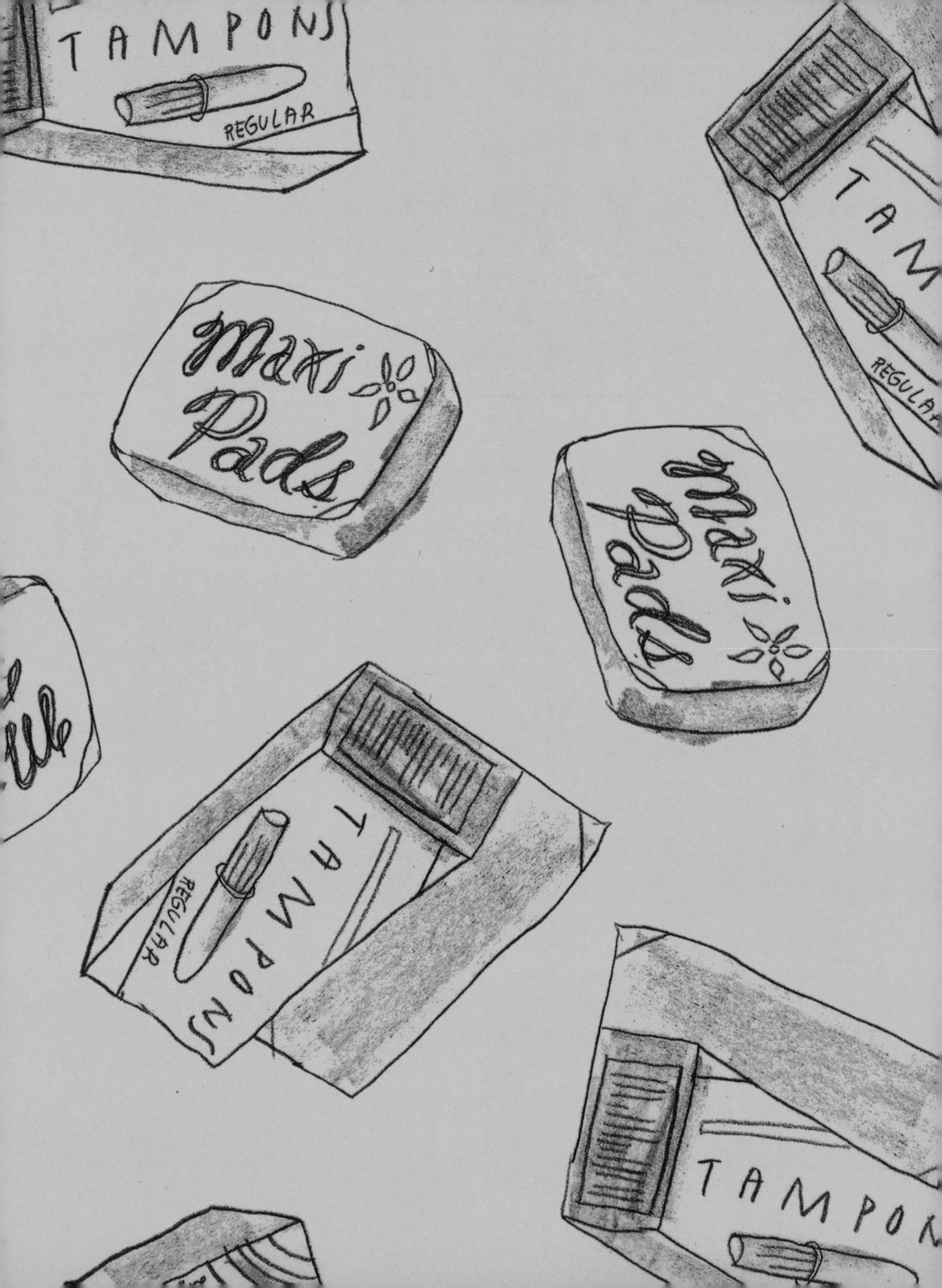
TAMPONS
REGULAR
Maxi Pads
Maxi Pads
TAMPONS
REGULAR

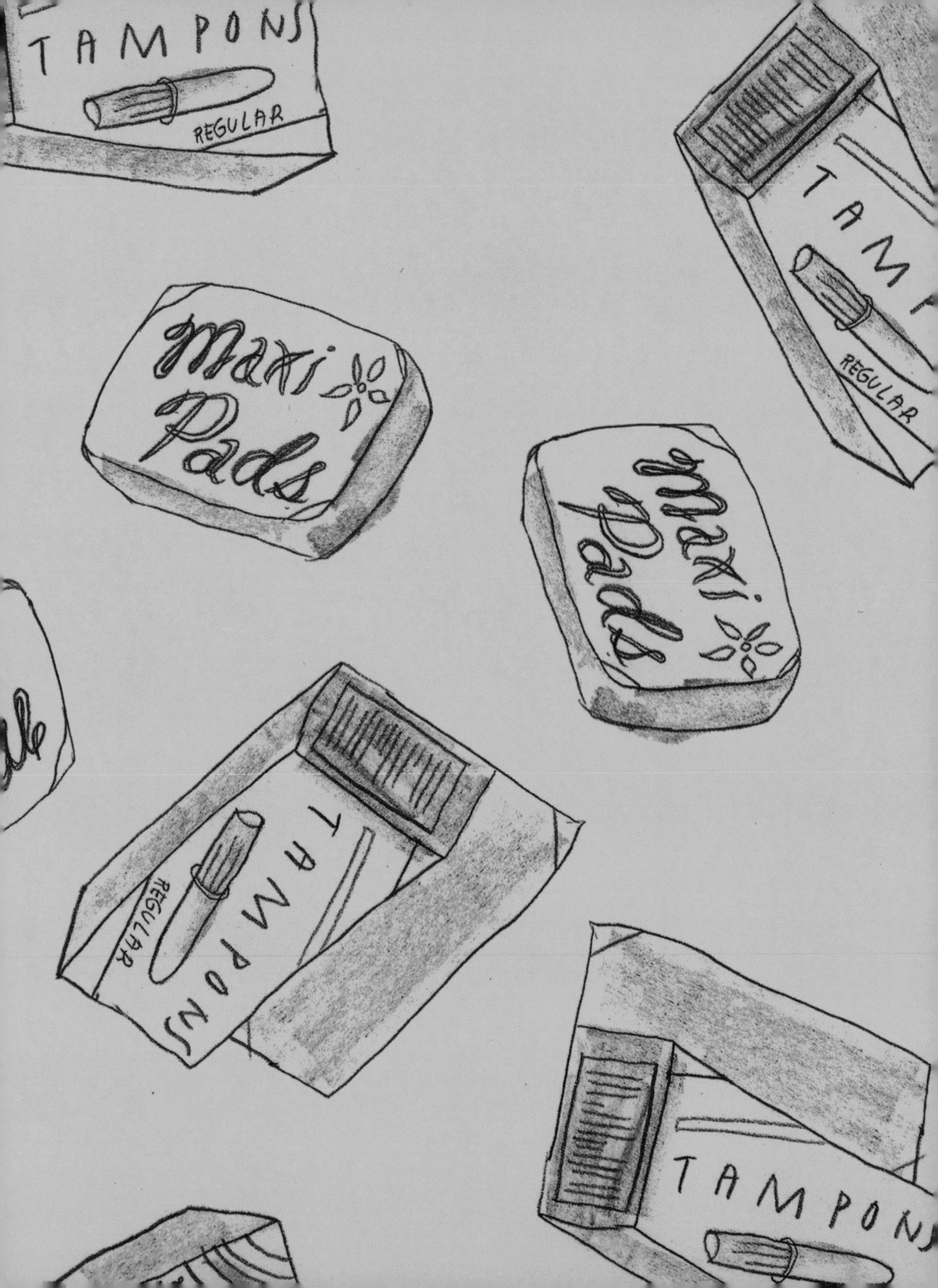
TAMPONS
REGULAR
Maxi Pads
Maxi Pads
TAMPONS
REGULAR
TAMPONS
REGULAR
TAMPONS

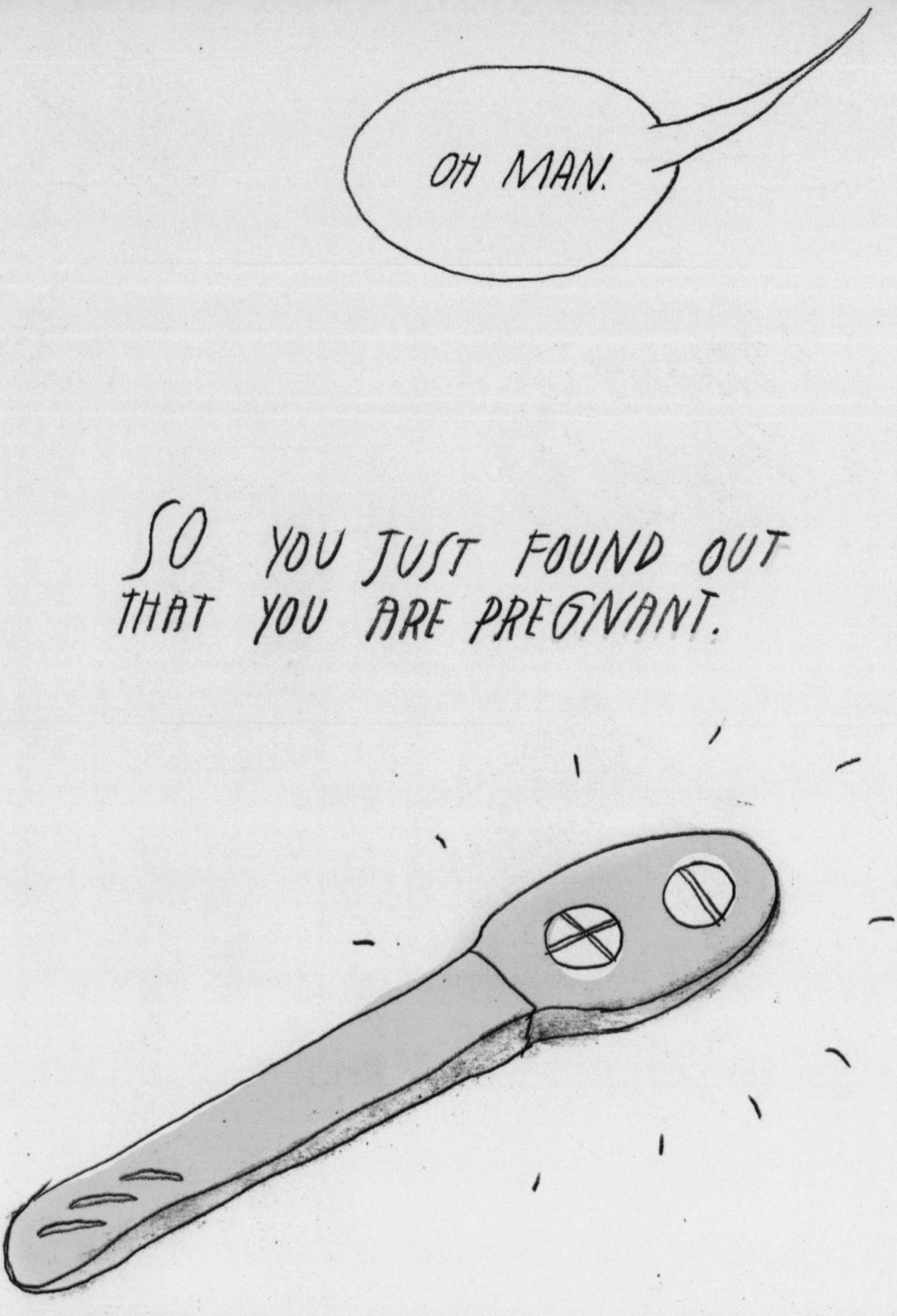
OH MAN.
SO YOU JUST FOUND OUT THAT YOU ARE PREGNANT.

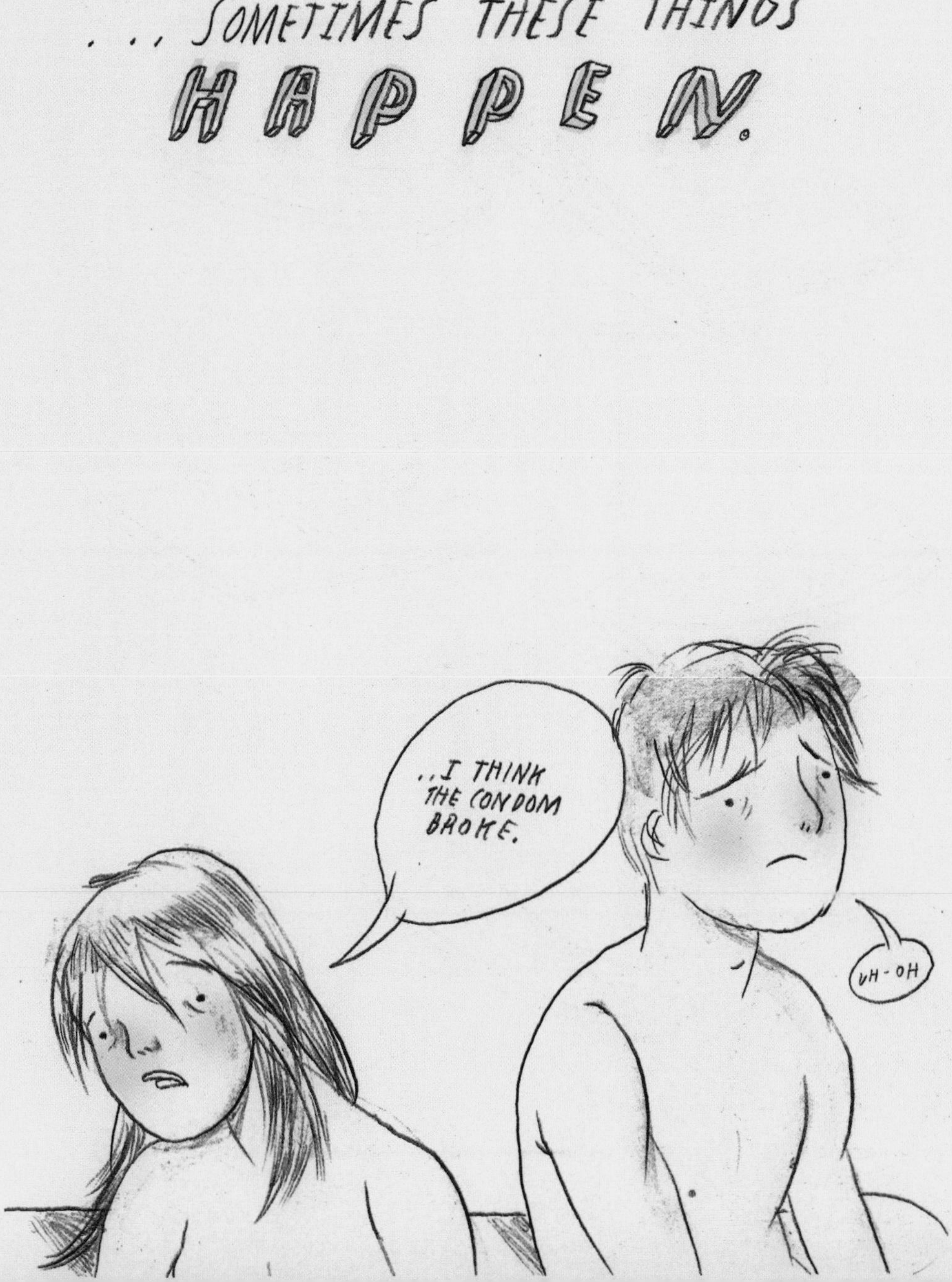
...SOMETIMES THESE THINGS
HAPPEN.
..I THINK THE CONDOM BROKE.
UH-OH

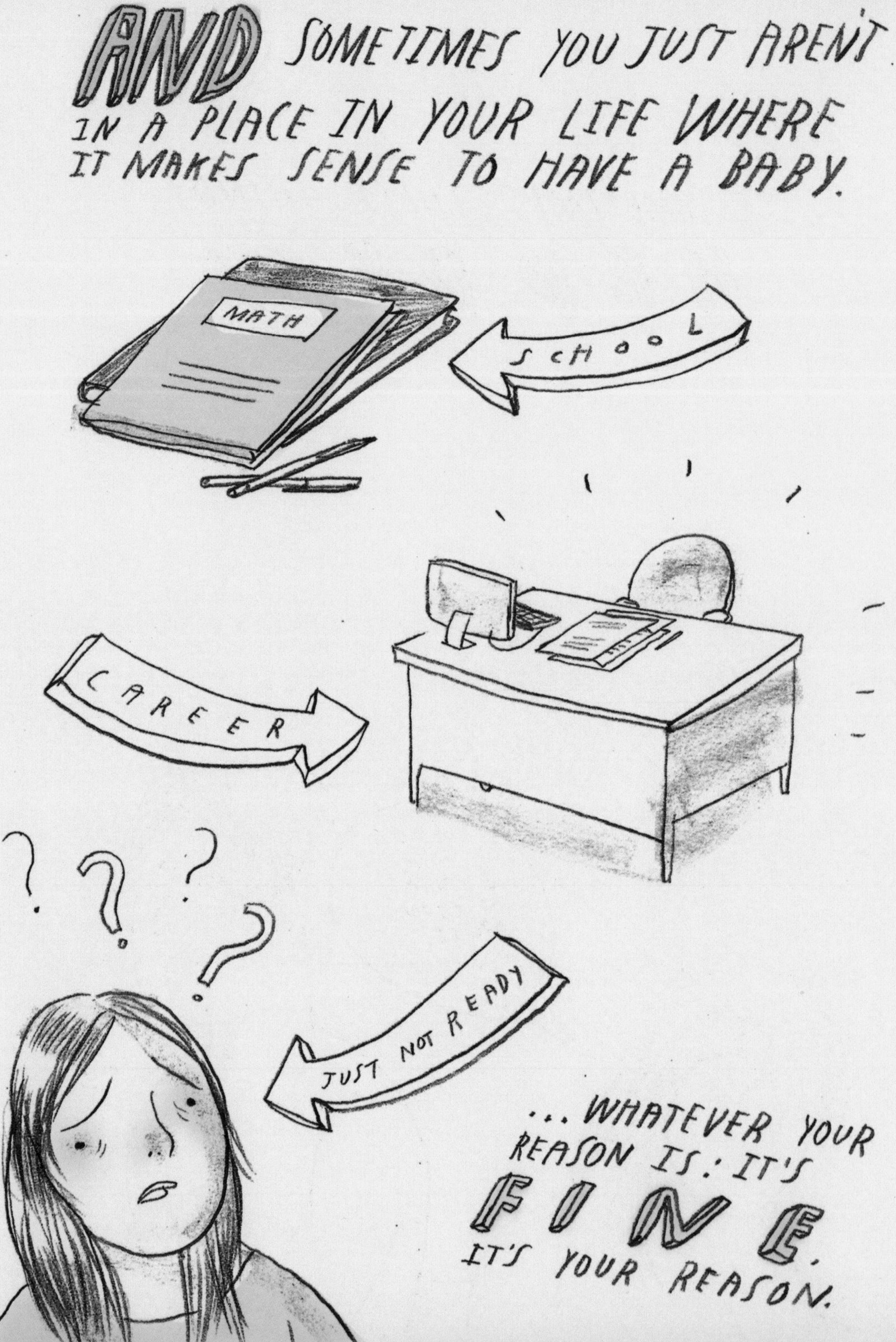
AND SOMETIMES YOU JUST AREN'T IN A PLACE IN YOUR LIFE WHERE IT MAKES SENSE TO HAVE A BABY.
MATH
SCHOOL
CAREER
JUST NOT READY
...WHATEVER YOUR REASON IS: IT'S FINE. IT'S YOUR REASON.

IF YOU HAVE AN "ACCIDENT,"
THERE IS A PILL YOU CAN TAKE UP
TO 120 HOURS AFTER THE INCIDENT.

THE SOONER YOU TAKE IT, THE
MORE EFFECTIVE IT IS. THIS IS
CALLED THE EMERGENCY CONTRACEPTION PILL,
AND YOU CAN BUY IT AT THE DRUGSTORE.

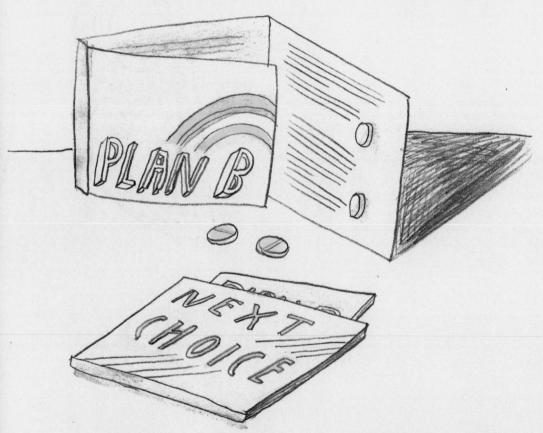

IT GENERALLY WORKS AND IS PRETTY EASY
TO TAKE, ALTHO THIS IS ONLY AN OPTION IF
YOU ACT RIGHT AWAY.

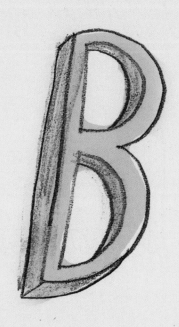

T

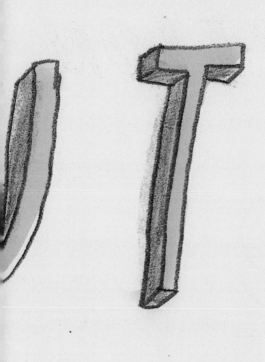

IF YOU FIND OUT THAT YOU ARE PREGNANT LATER ON (LIKE IF YOU MISS YOUR PERIOD..), THEN YOU MAY DECIDE TO HAVE AN

ABORTION.

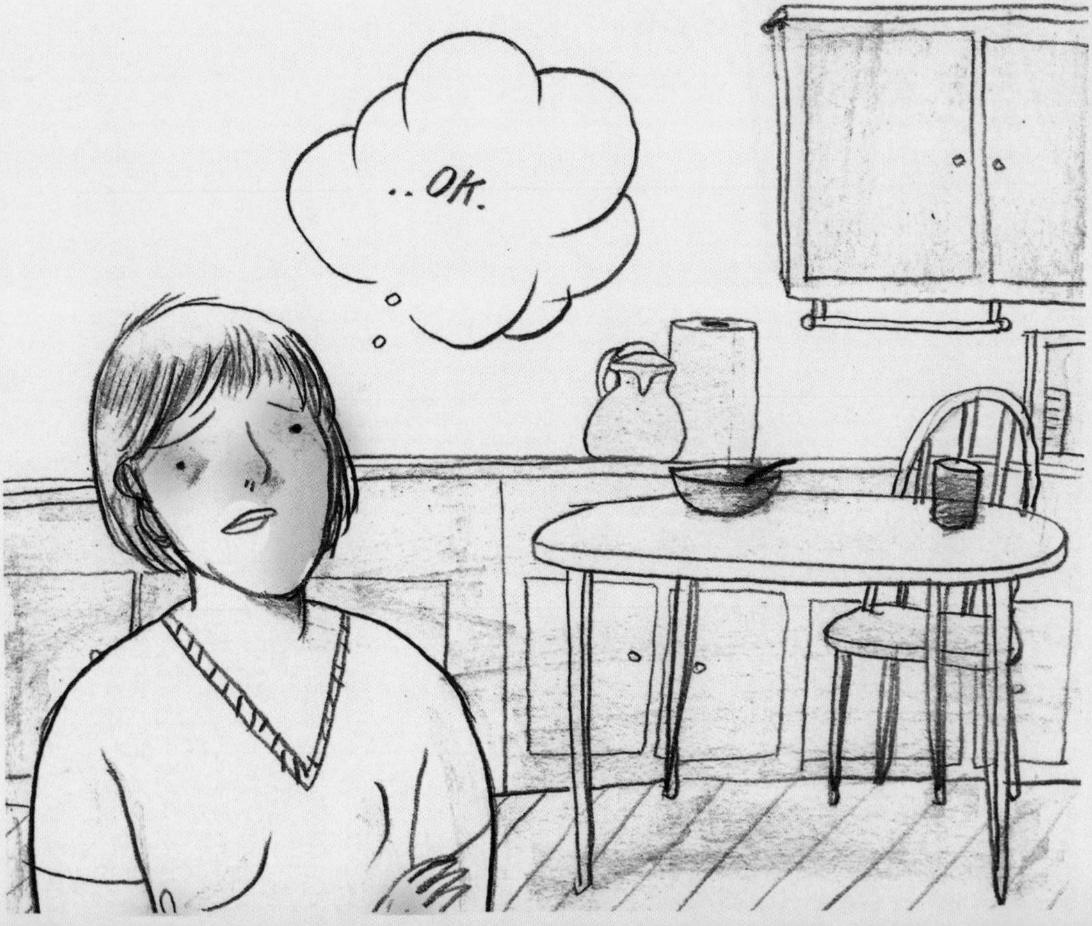
..OK.

WHETHER IT'S A COMPLICATED DECISION OR A NO-BRAINER; WHETHER YOU HAVE A PARTNER OR YOU DON'T; WHETHER YOU HAVE AN AWESOME RELATIONSHIP WITH YOUR FAMILY OR A LESS-THAN-AWESOME ONE... THE IMPORTANT THING TO REMEMBER IS THAT THE FINAL DECISION IS **YOURS**, AND NO ONE IS ALLOWED TO TELL YOU WHAT TO DO. (DUH... IT'S **YOUR** BODY.)

I DON'T KNOW. I THINK YOU'RE MAKING A MISTAKE
...AND THAT IS WHY YOU CAN GO SCREW.

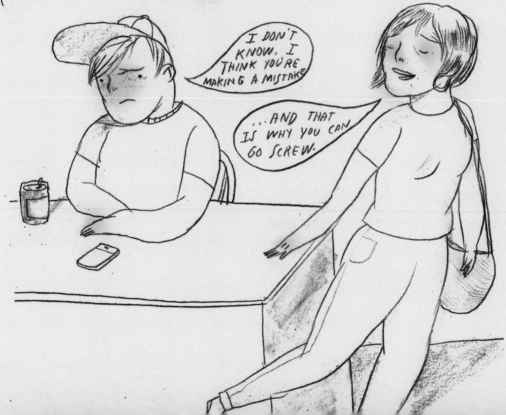

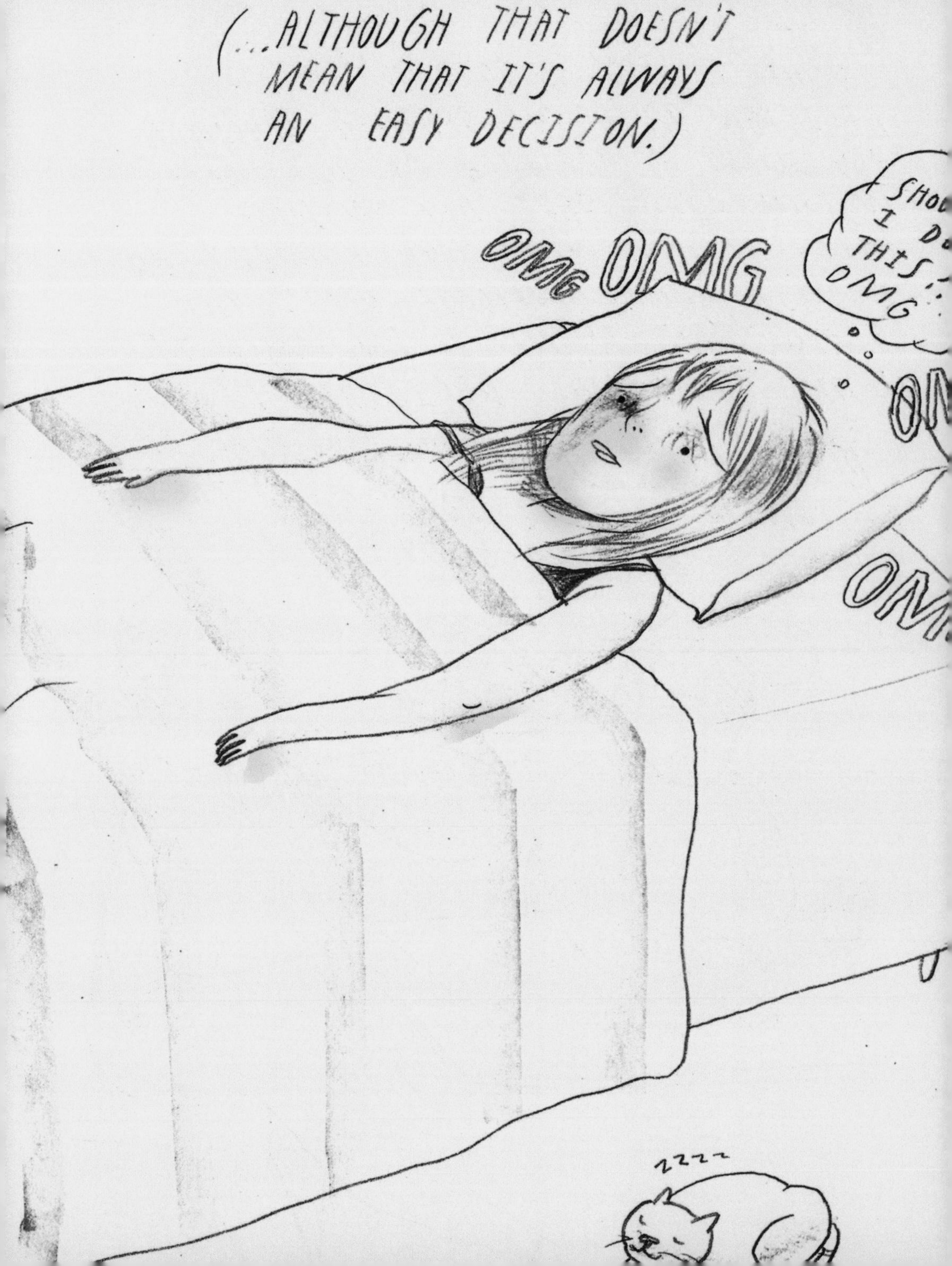
(...ALTHOUGH THAT DOESN'T MEAN THAT IT'S ALWAYS AN EASY DECISION.)
OMG OMG
THIS... OMG
OMG
OMG
ZZZZ

FEB 2014
1
2
3
4
5
6
7
8
9
10
11
12

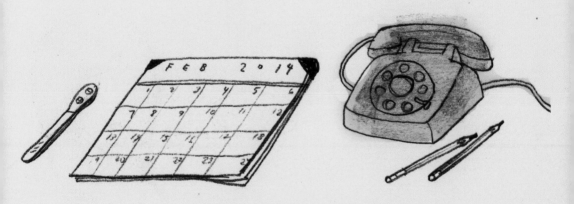

...SO HERE WE ARE.

IF IT MAKES YOU FEEL BETTER, LET'S TALK ABOUT TWO DIFFERENT GIRLS WHO WENT THROUGH TWO DIFFERENT ABORTIONS. THERE ARE A ZILLION GIRLS WHO GO THROUGH THIS, BUT DESPITE KNOWING... IT CAN STILL FEEL VERY LONELY AT TIMES.

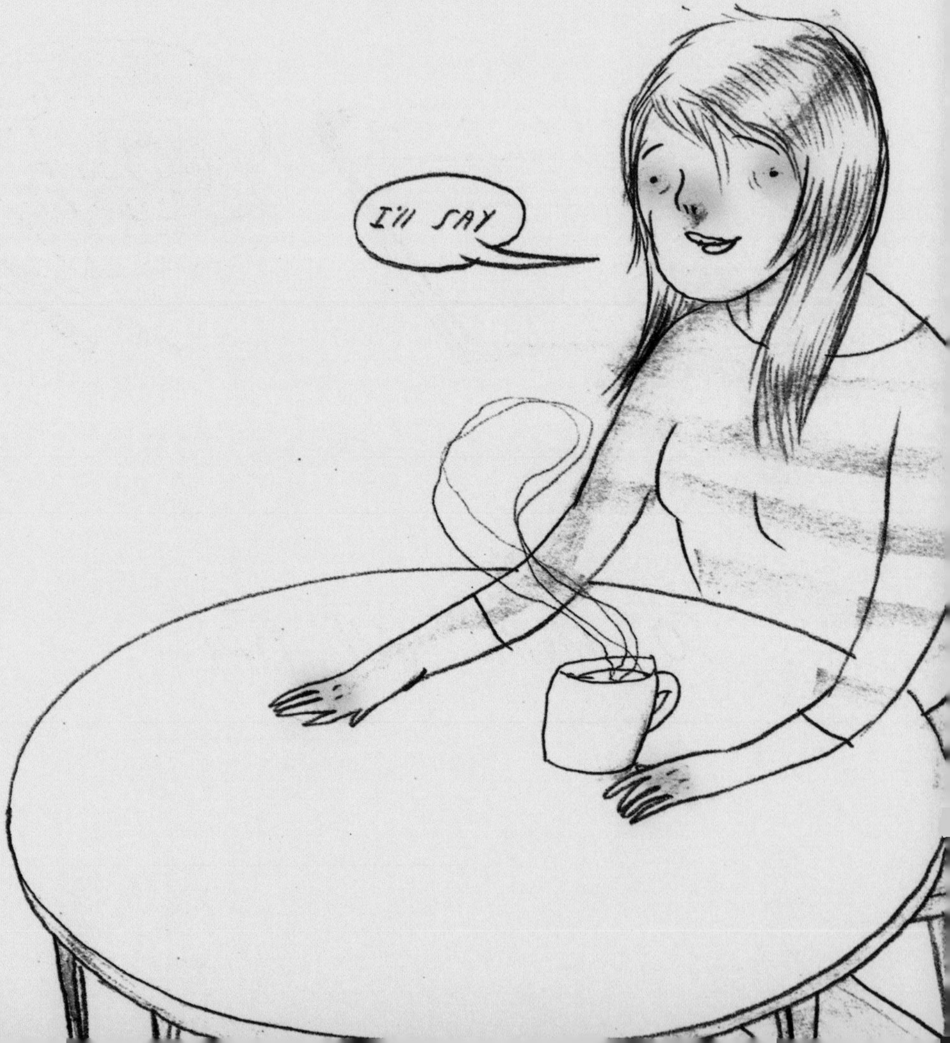
I'LL SAY

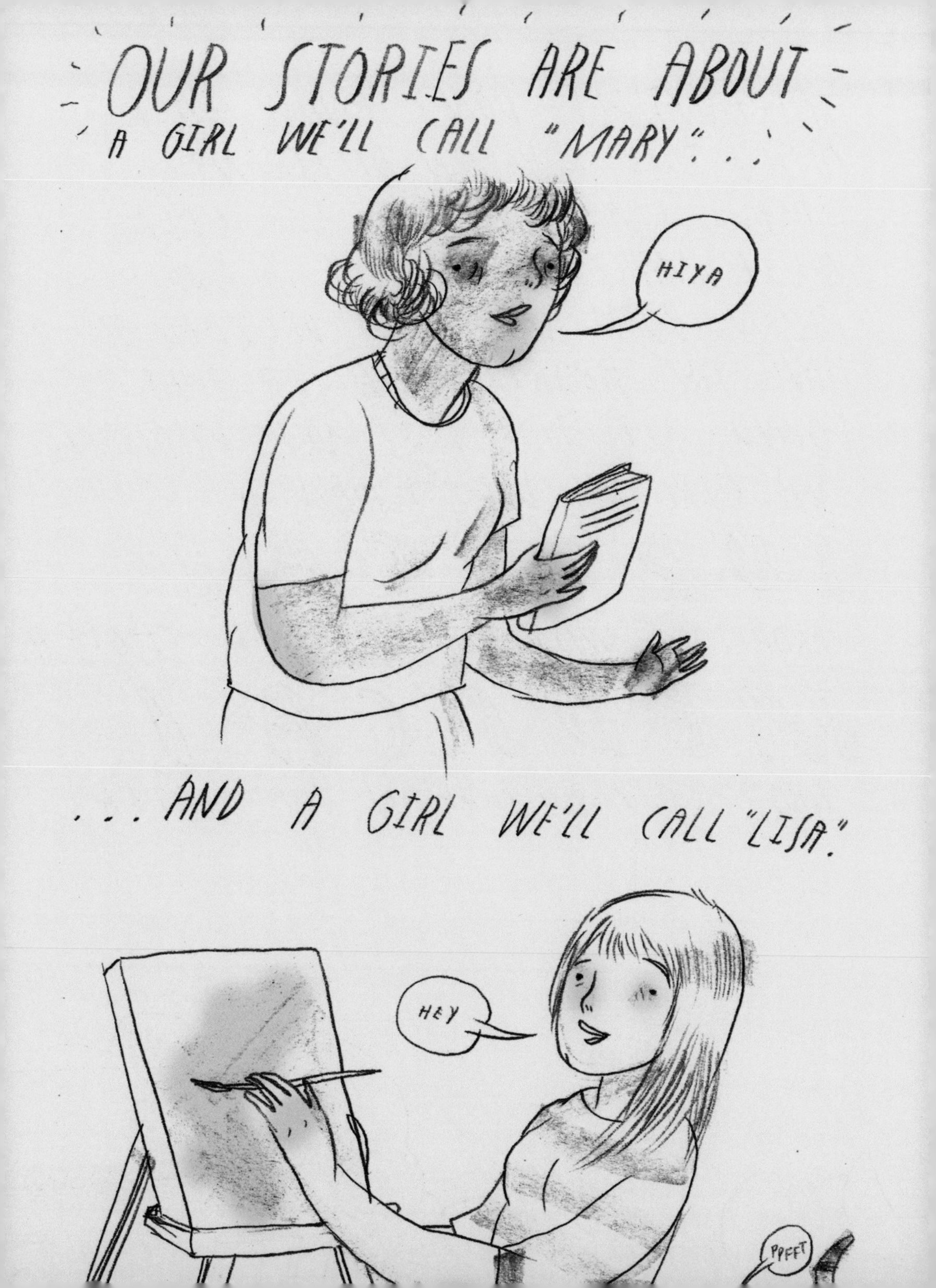
OUR STORIES ARE ABOUT
A GIRL WE'LL CALL "MARY"...
HIYA
...AND A GIRL WE'LL CALL "LISA."
HEY
PPFFT

THESE GIRLS DON'T KNOW EACH OTHER. THEY LIVE IN DIFFERENT PLACES: LISA LIVES IN THE CITY WHILE MARY LIVES IN A SMALL TOWN. BOTH OF THEM DECIDED TO HAVE AN ABORTION AFTER THEY FOUND OUT THAT THEY WERE PREGNANT. ONE GIRL DECIDED TO HAVE A

SURGICAL

ABORTION, WHILE THE OTHER CHOSE A

MEDICAL

ABORTION (BUT MORE ON THAT LATER).

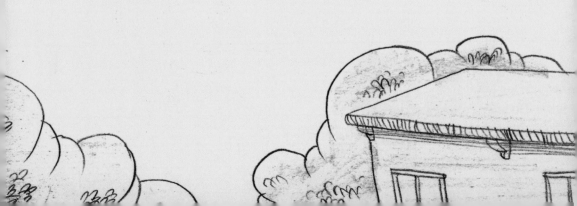

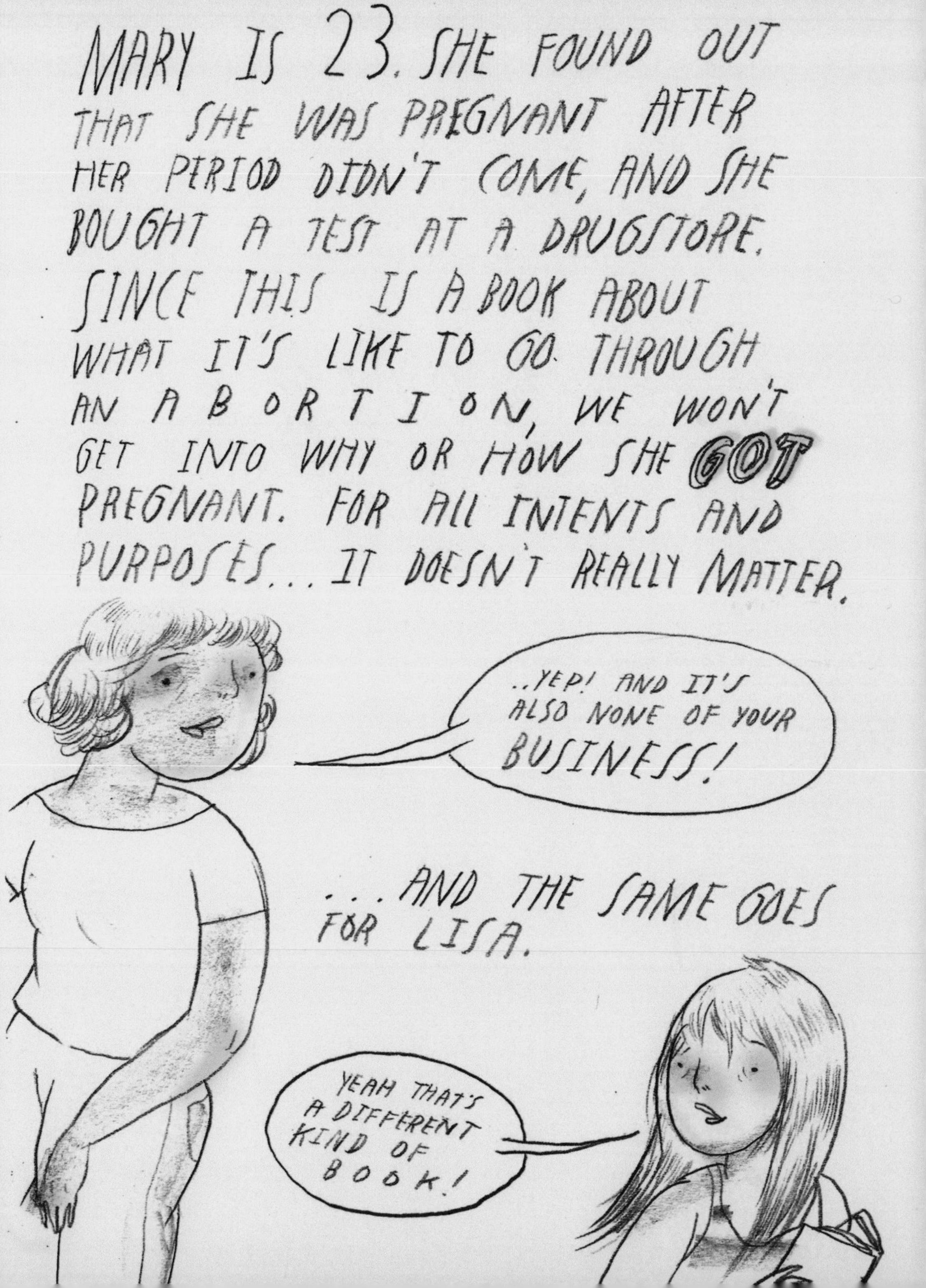
MARY IS 23. SHE FOUND OUT THAT SHE WAS PREGNANT AFTER HER PERIOD DIDN'T COME, AND SHE BOUGHT A TEST AT A DRUGSTORE. SINCE THIS IS A BOOK ABOUT WHAT IT'S LIKE TO GO THROUGH AN A B O R T I O N, WE WON'T GET INTO WHY OR HOW SHE GOT PREGNANT. FOR ALL INTENTS AND PURPOSES... IT DOESN'T REALLY MATTER.
..YEP! AND IT'S ALSO NONE OF YOUR BUSINESS!
...AND THE SAME GOES FOR LISA.
YEAH THAT'S A DIFFERENT KIND OF B O O K!

THE **POINT** IS:
BOTH GIRLS CHOSE TO GO
THROUGH THE SAME THING,
NO MATTER HOW THEY GOT
THERE.

LISA IS 31. SHE DECIDED TO GO TO HER DOCTOR AND TAKE A PREGNANCY TEST AFTER SHE FELT SICK FOR A FEW DAYS BEFORE HER PERIOD. SINCE HER PERIODS HAD NEVER BEEN REGULAR, SHE WASN'T SURE IF SHE WAS LATE. BEFORE HER APPOINTMENT, SHE ALSO TOOK A HOME TEST (OR FIVE).

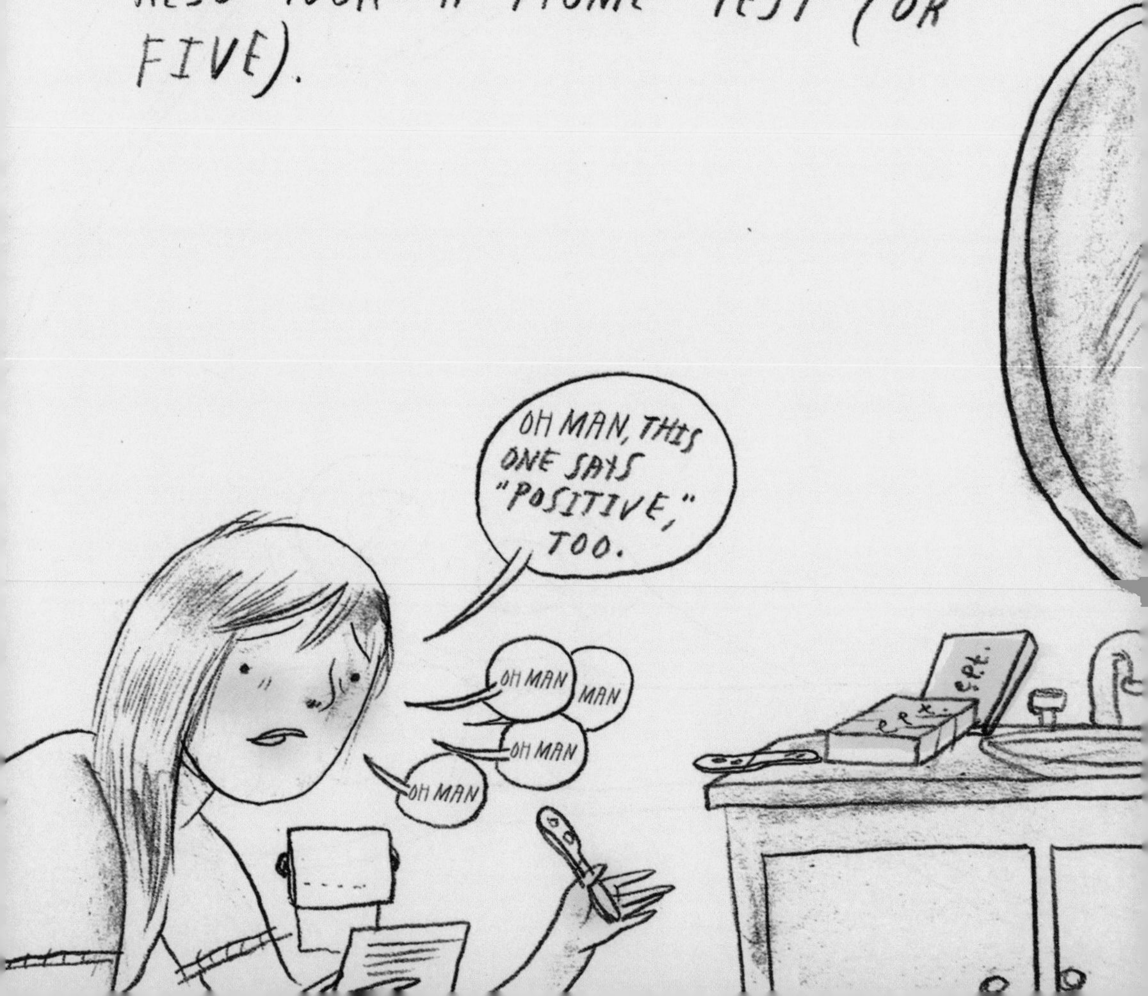
OH MAN, THIS ONE SAYS "POSITIVE," TOO.
OH MAN
MAN
OH MAN
OH MAN

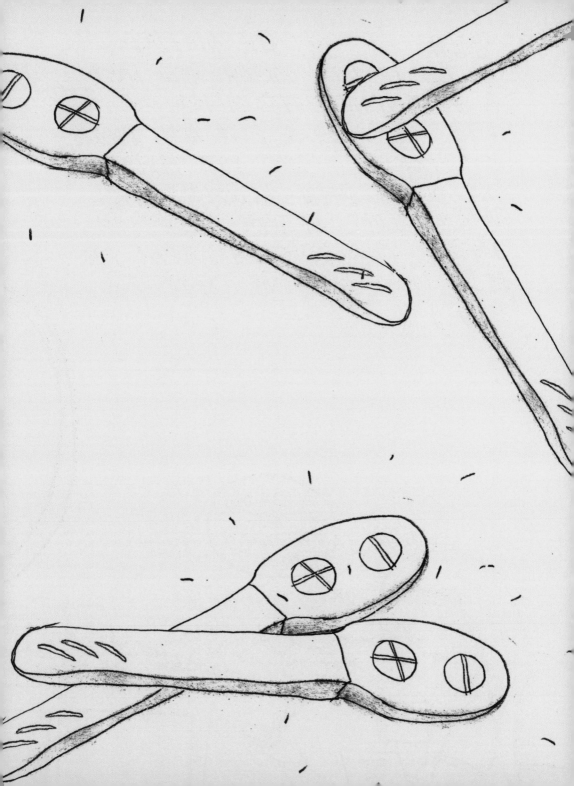

SOMETIMES HAVING
AN **ABORTION** IS
A NO-BRAINER, SOMETIMES
IT'S NOT. BUT FOR THE TIME BEING,
WE WON'T GET INTO ALL OF THAT.

OUR STORY REALLY BEGINS

N O W,

WHEN BOTH GIRLS DECIDE (FOR
DIFFERENT, PERSONAL REASONS)
TO GO AHEAD AND HAVE AN ABORTION.

KNOWING THAT YOU ARE PREGNANT WHEN YOU DIDN'T EXPECT OR WANT TO BE CAN BE SCARY. YOU HAVE TO MAKE APPOINTMENTS AND FIGURE STUFF OUT FAIRLY QUICKLY. WHICH CAN BE HARD TO DO IF YOU'RE SCARED. BUT FIRST TAKE A DEEP BREATH, AND TELL YOURSELF THAT EVERYTHING IS GOING TO BE OK. BECAUSE THAT WILL HELP YOU GET THRU THE NEXT STEPS.

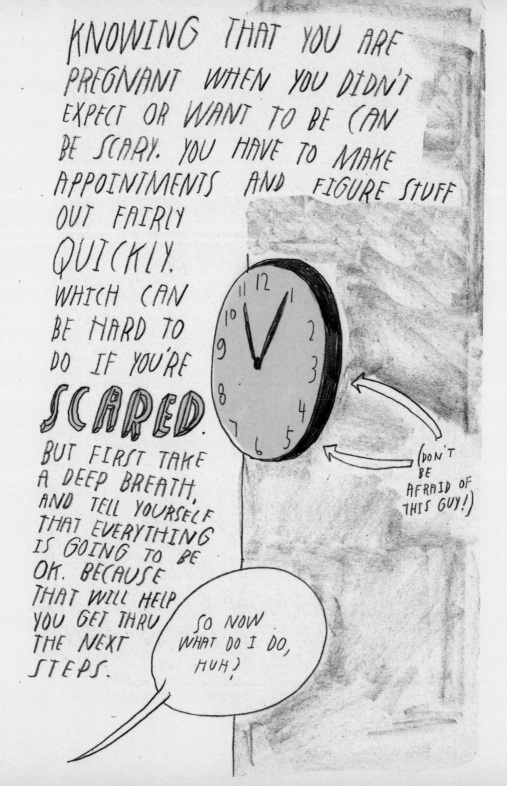

(DON'T BE AFRAID OF THIS GUY!)

SO NOW WHAT DO I DO, HUH?

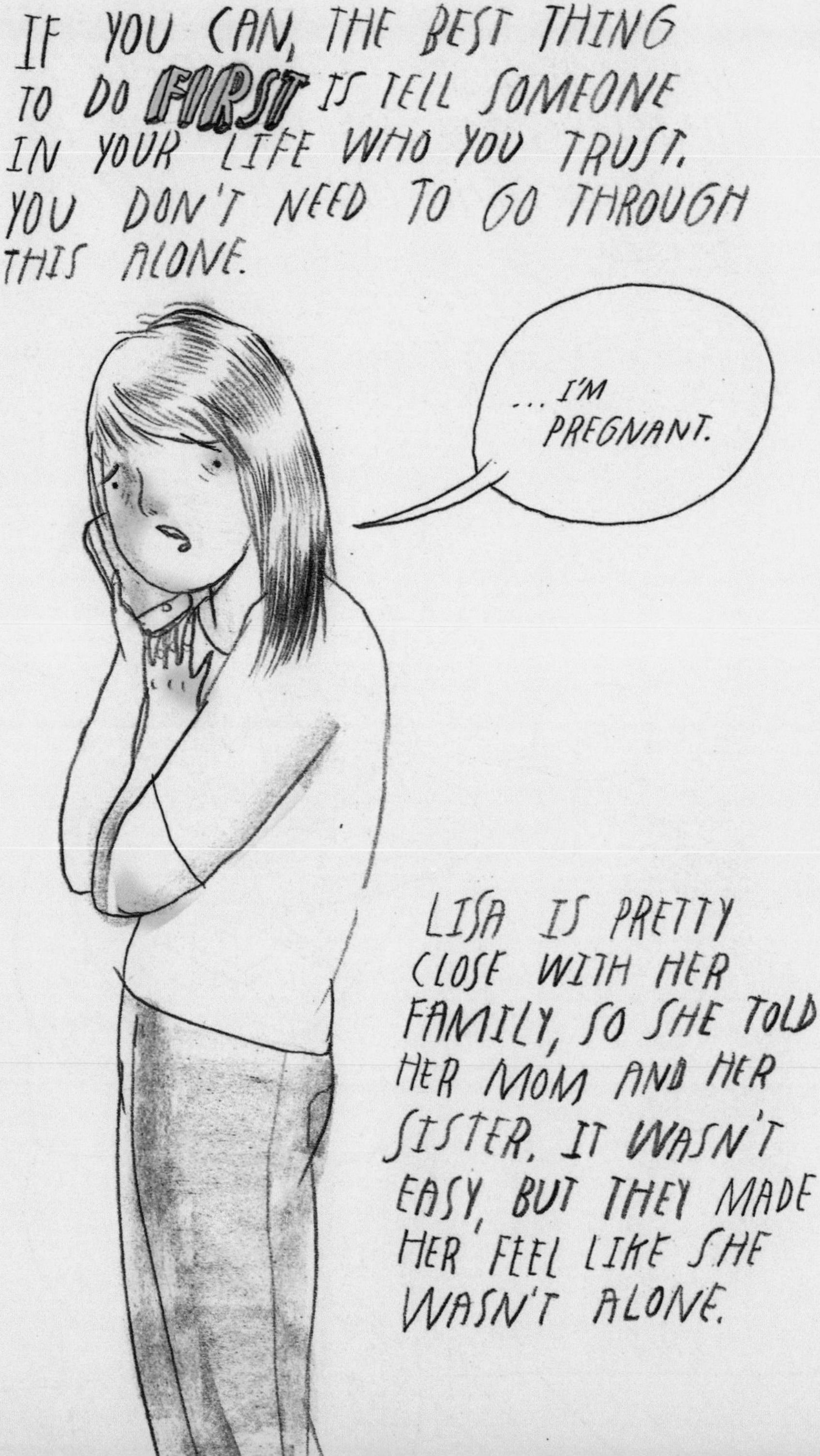

IF YOU CAN, THE BEST THING TO DO **FIRST** IS TELL SOMEONE IN YOUR LIFE WHO YOU TRUST. YOU DON'T NEED TO GO THROUGH THIS ALONE.

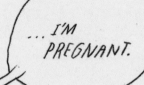

... I'M PREGNANT.

LISA IS PRETTY CLOSE WITH HER FAMILY, SO SHE TOLD HER MOM AND HER SISTER. IT WASN'T EASY, BUT THEY MADE HER FEEL LIKE SHE WASN'T ALONE.

MARY ISN'T AS CLOSE TO HER FAMILY, SO SHE PREFERRED NOT TO TELL THEM. SHE TOLD HER BEST FRIEND.

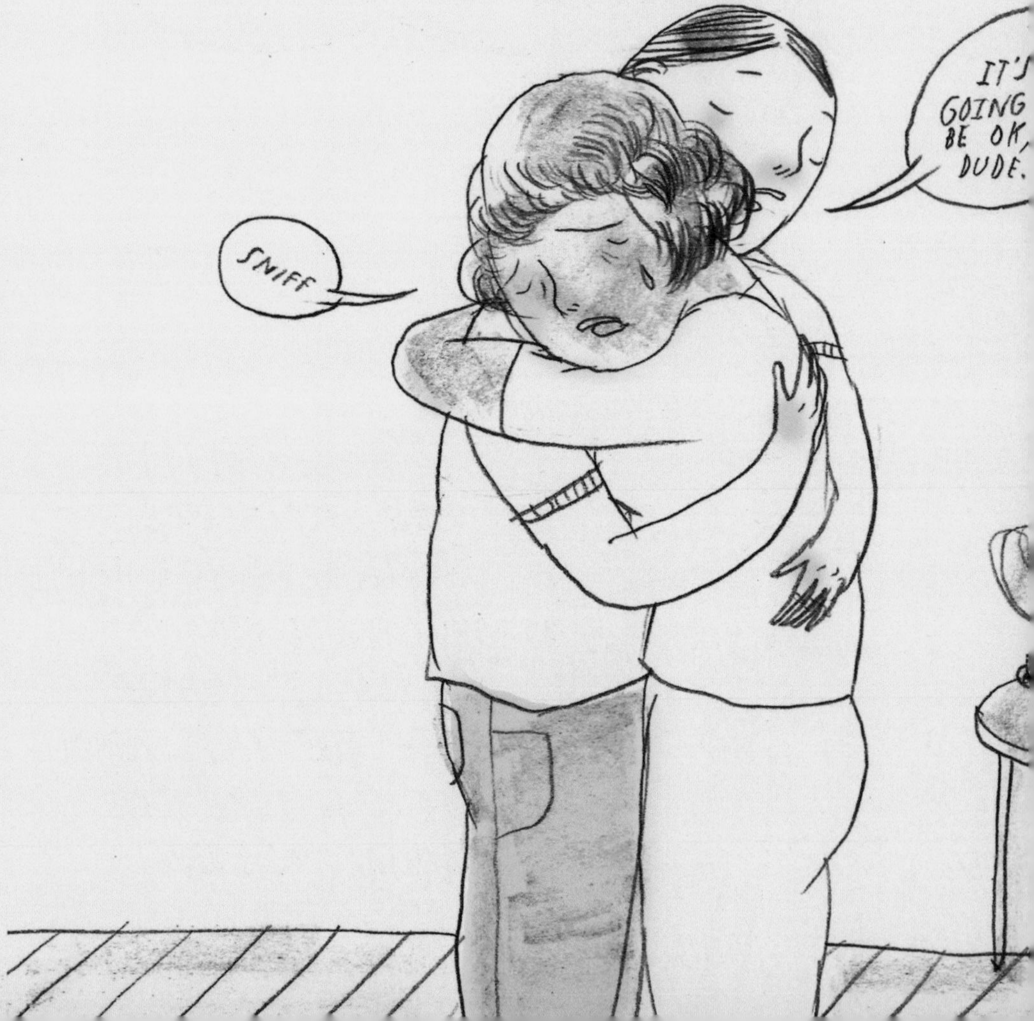
SNIFF
IT'S GOING BE OK, DUDE.

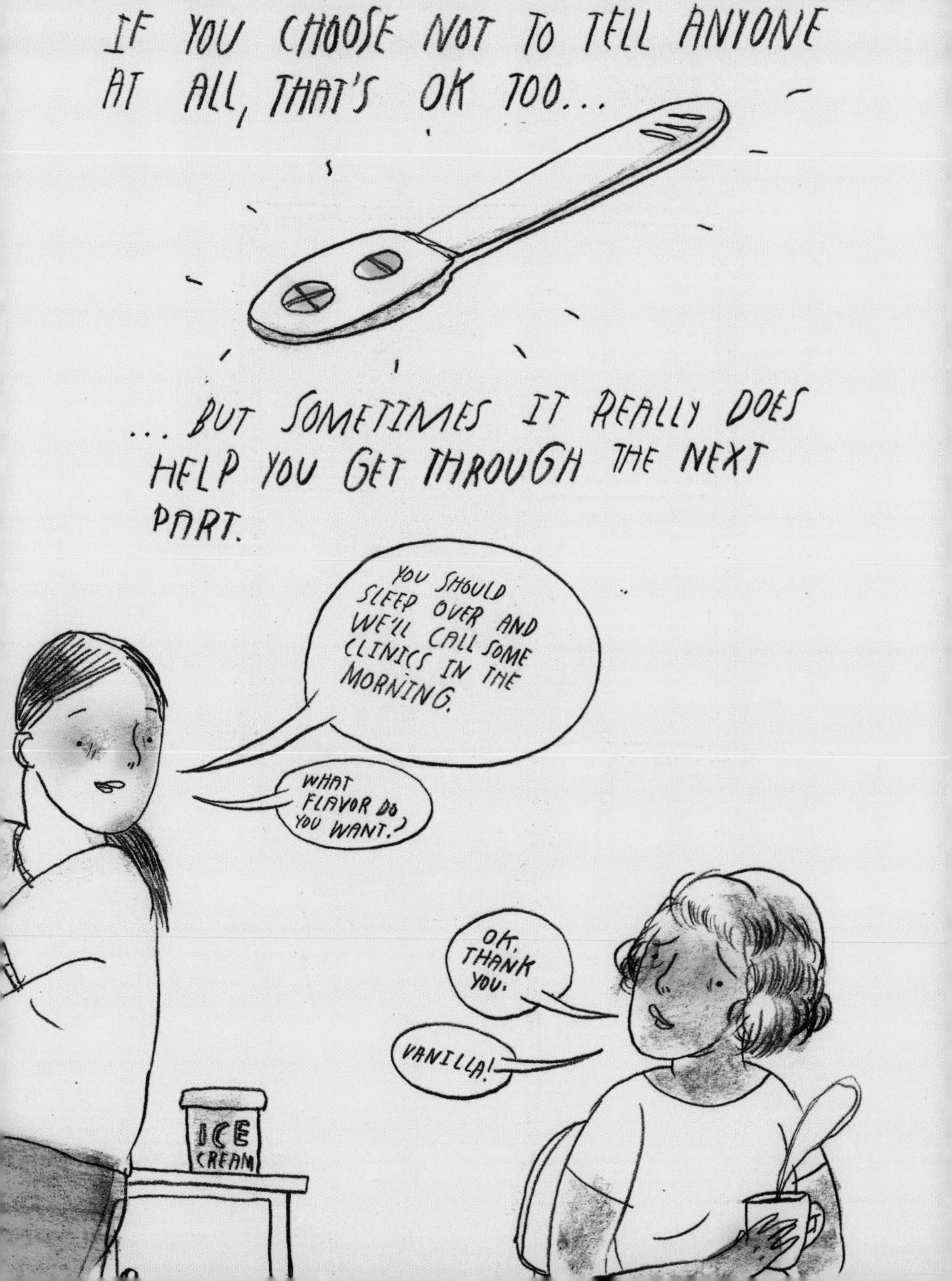
IF YOU CHOOSE NOT TO TELL ANYONE AT ALL, THAT'S OK TOO...
...BUT SOMETIMES IT REALLY DOES HELP YOU GET THROUGH THE NEXT PART.
YOU SHOULD SLEEP OVER AND WE'LL CALL SOME CLINICS IN THE MORNING.
WHAT FLAVOR DO YOU WANT?
OK. THANK YOU.
VANILLA!
ICE CREAM

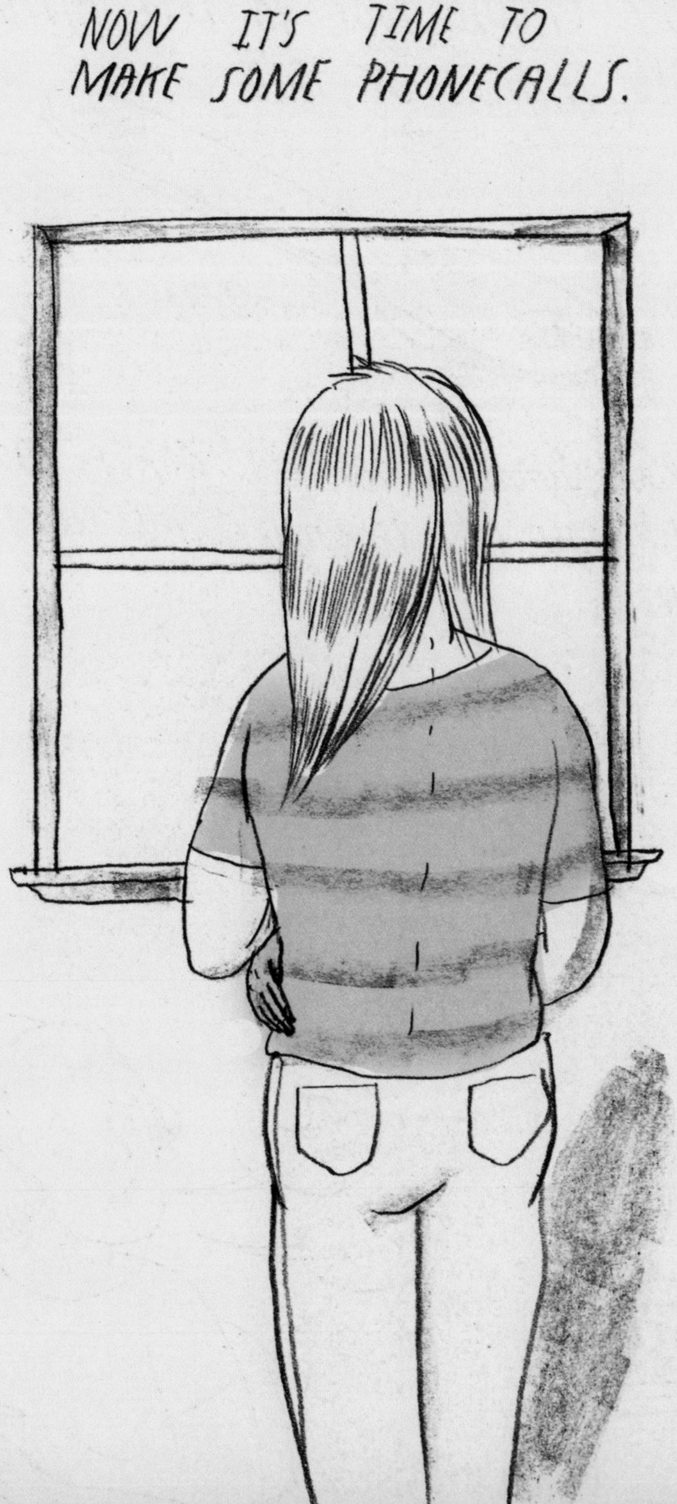
NOW IT'S TIME TO MAKE SOME PHONECALLS.

THERE ARE **THREE**

THINGS TO CONSIDER RIGHT
AWAY, ONCE YOU'VE MADE
THE DECISION TO HAVE AN
ABORTION.

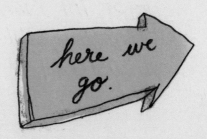
here we go.

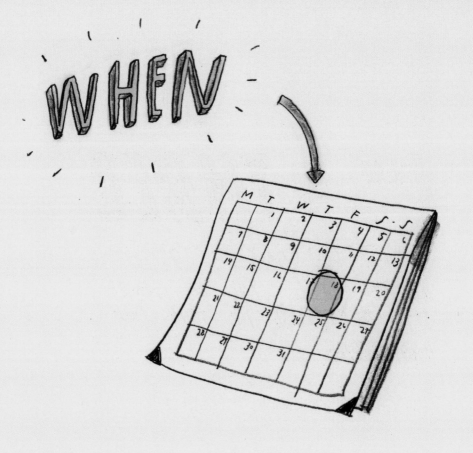

...THIS IS THE TIME-SENSITIVE PART. THE SOONER AFTER YOU FIND OUT, THE EASIER IT WILL BE ON YA (IN SOME WAYS)!

. . . CLINIC? AT HOME (THIS ONE SHALL BE EXPLAINED LATER!)?

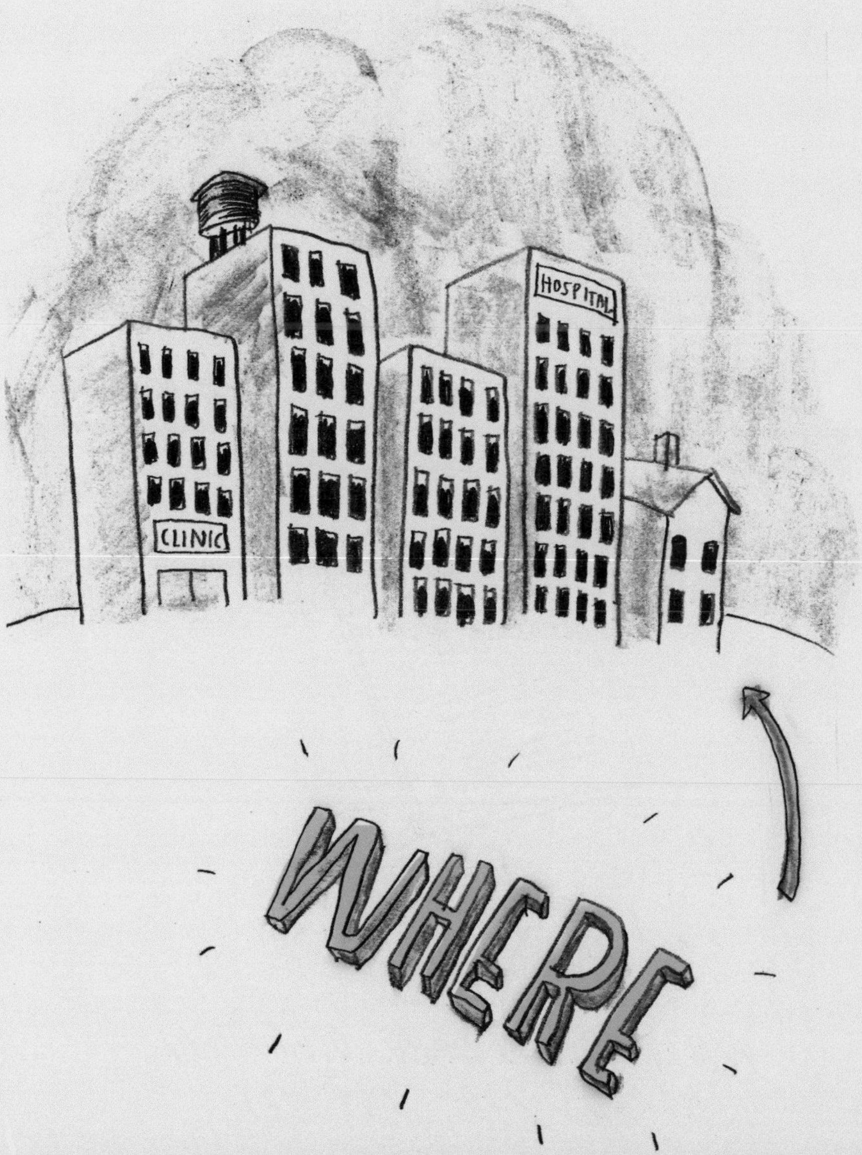
HOSPITAL
CLINIC
WHERE

WHAT
Surgical abortion + YOU
MEDICAL ABORTION
WHAT TO EXPECT

. . . "WAIT: THERE ARE DIFFERENT KINDS???" OH YES.

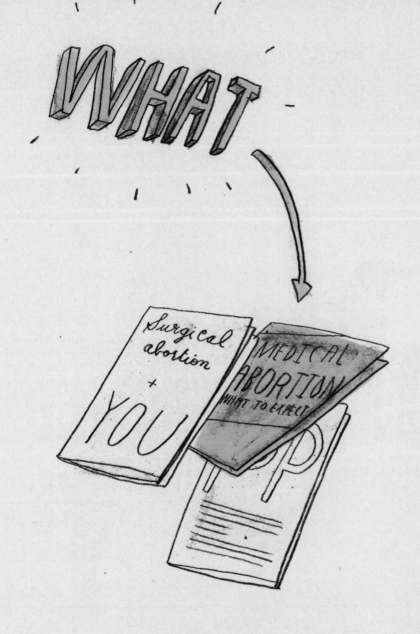

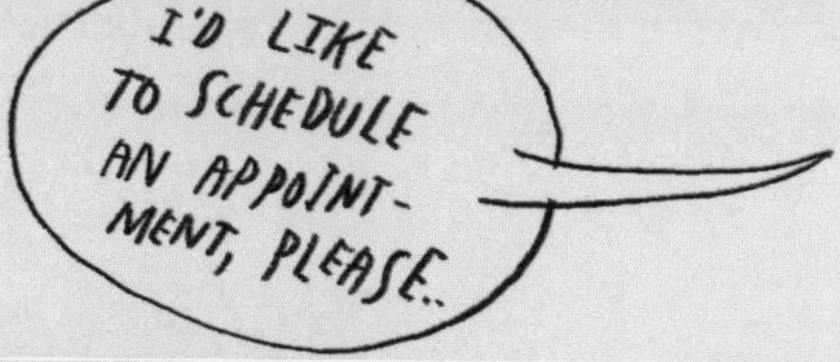
I'D LIKE TO SCHEDULE AN APPOINTMENT, PLEASE..

"WHERE" "WHEN" AND "WHAT"

ARE TIME SENSITIVE BECAUSE THE OPTIONS CHANGE THE LONGER YOU WAIT.* EVEN THOUGH IT MAY ALL FEEL VERY OVERWHELMING, PICKING UP THE PHONE AND MAKING A CALL TO SCHEDULE AN APPOINTMENT AS SOON AS POSSIBLE IS IMPORTANT. IF YOU HAVE A FRIEND OR FAMILY MEMBER WHO CAN BE WITH YOU WHILE YOU MAKE THE CALL, THAT'S EVEN BETTER!

* (THE SAFEST TIME TO HAVE AN ABORTION IS DURING WHAT THEY CALL THE "*first trimester*" — OR UP TO WEEK TWELVE OF A PREGNANCY. ABORTIONS AFTER THIS BECOME MORE COMPLEX AND CAN POSE RISKS TO THE WOMAN.)

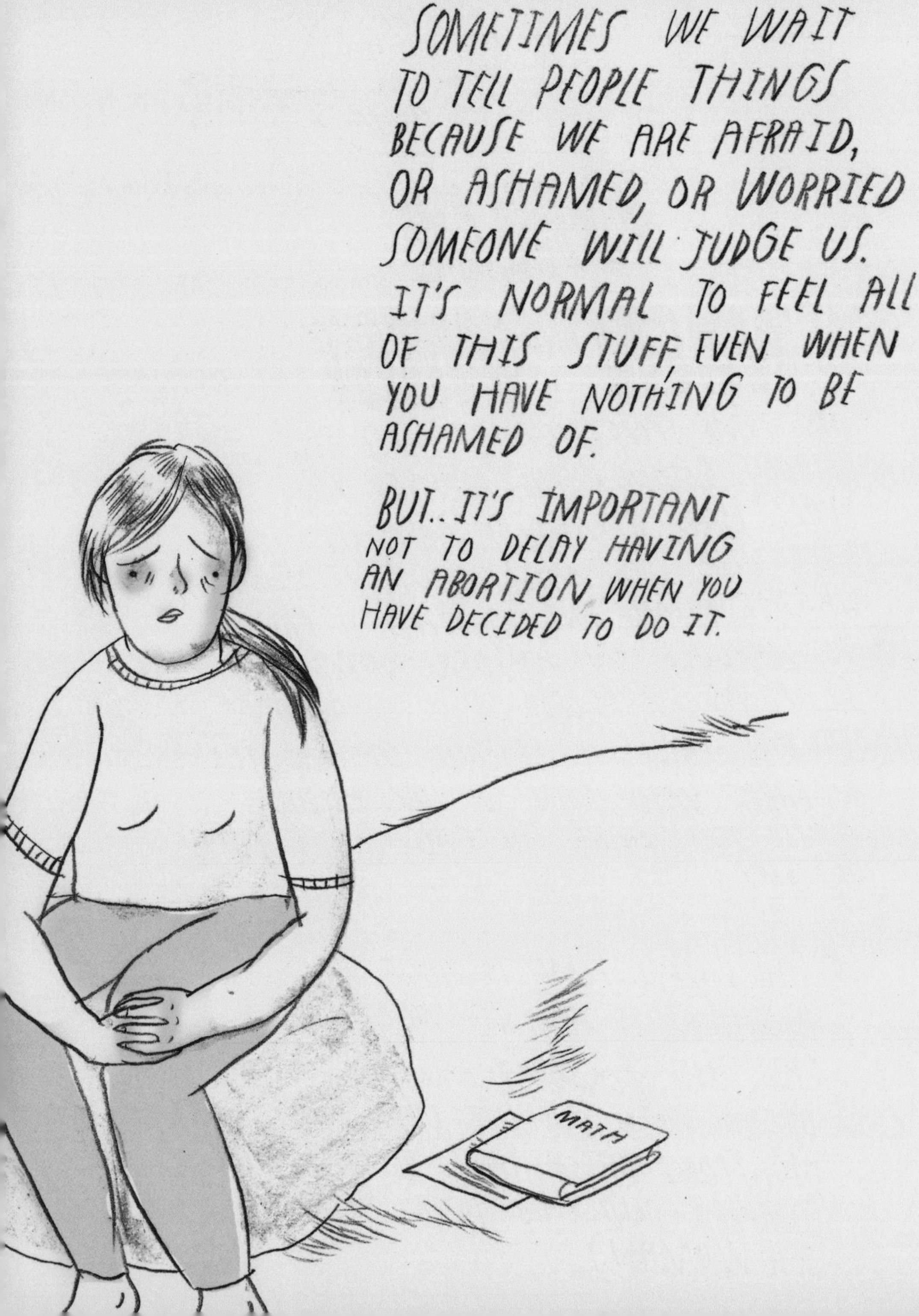
SOMETIMES WE WAIT TO TELL PEOPLE THINGS BECAUSE WE ARE AFRAID, OR ASHAMED, OR WORRIED SOMEONE WILL JUDGE US. IT'S NORMAL TO FEEL ALL OF THIS STUFF, EVEN WHEN YOU HAVE NOTHING TO BE ASHAMED OF.
BUT.. IT'S IMPORTANT NOT TO DELAY HAVING AN ABORTION WHEN YOU HAVE DECIDED TO DO IT.
MATH

ALMOST ALL ABORTIONS (IN THE U.S.A.!) TAKE PLACE IN A CLINIC.

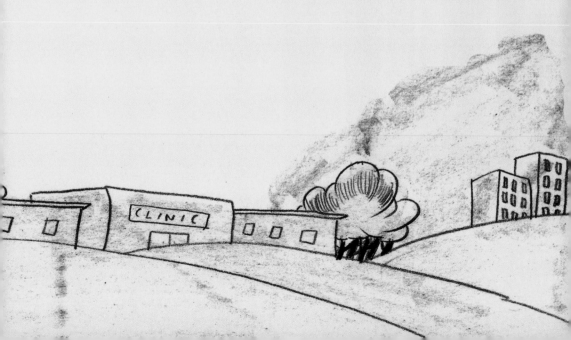

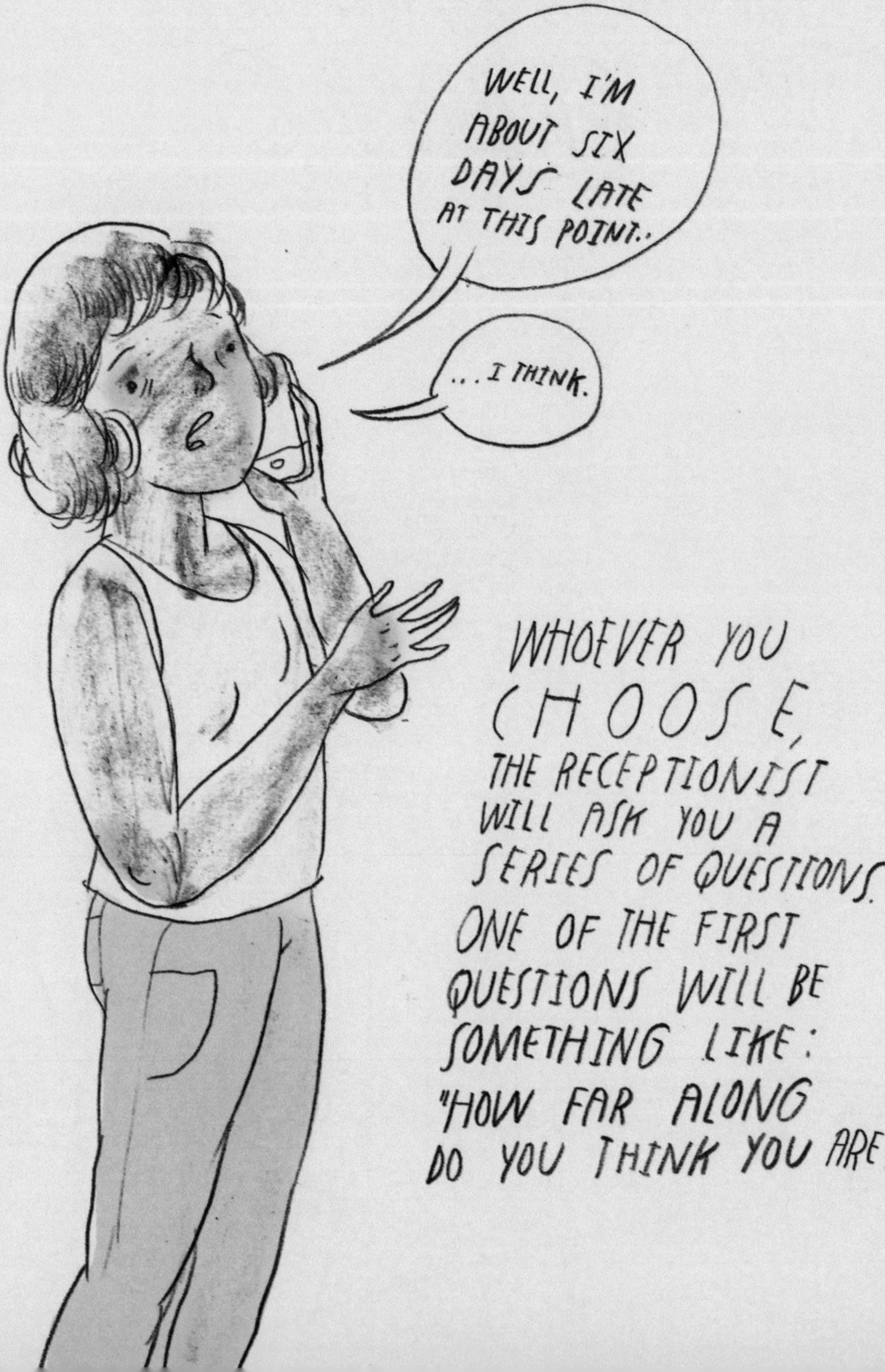
WELL, I'M ABOUT SIX DAYS LATE AT THIS POINT..
...I THINK.
WHOEVER YOU CHOOSE, THE RECEPTIONIST WILL ASK YOU A SERIES OF QUESTIONS. ONE OF THE FIRST QUESTIONS WILL BE SOMETHING LIKE: "HOW FAR ALONG DO YOU THINK YOU ARE?"

TAMPAX
Light

TAMPONS
REGULAR

Maxi
Pads

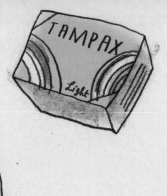

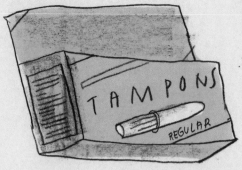

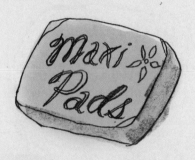

IT'S **OK** IF YOU DON'T KNOW THE EXACT ANSWER TO THIS. TRY TO REMEMBER THE DATE OF YOUR LAST PERIOD, HOW MANY DAYS LATE YOU ARE, AND THE NURSE WILL HELP DETERMINE HOW MANY WEEKS PREGNANT YOU ARE. THEN SHE (OR HE) CAN MAKE A PLAN WITH YOU ABOUT **WHAT** KIND OF ABORTION YOU SHOULD HAVE.

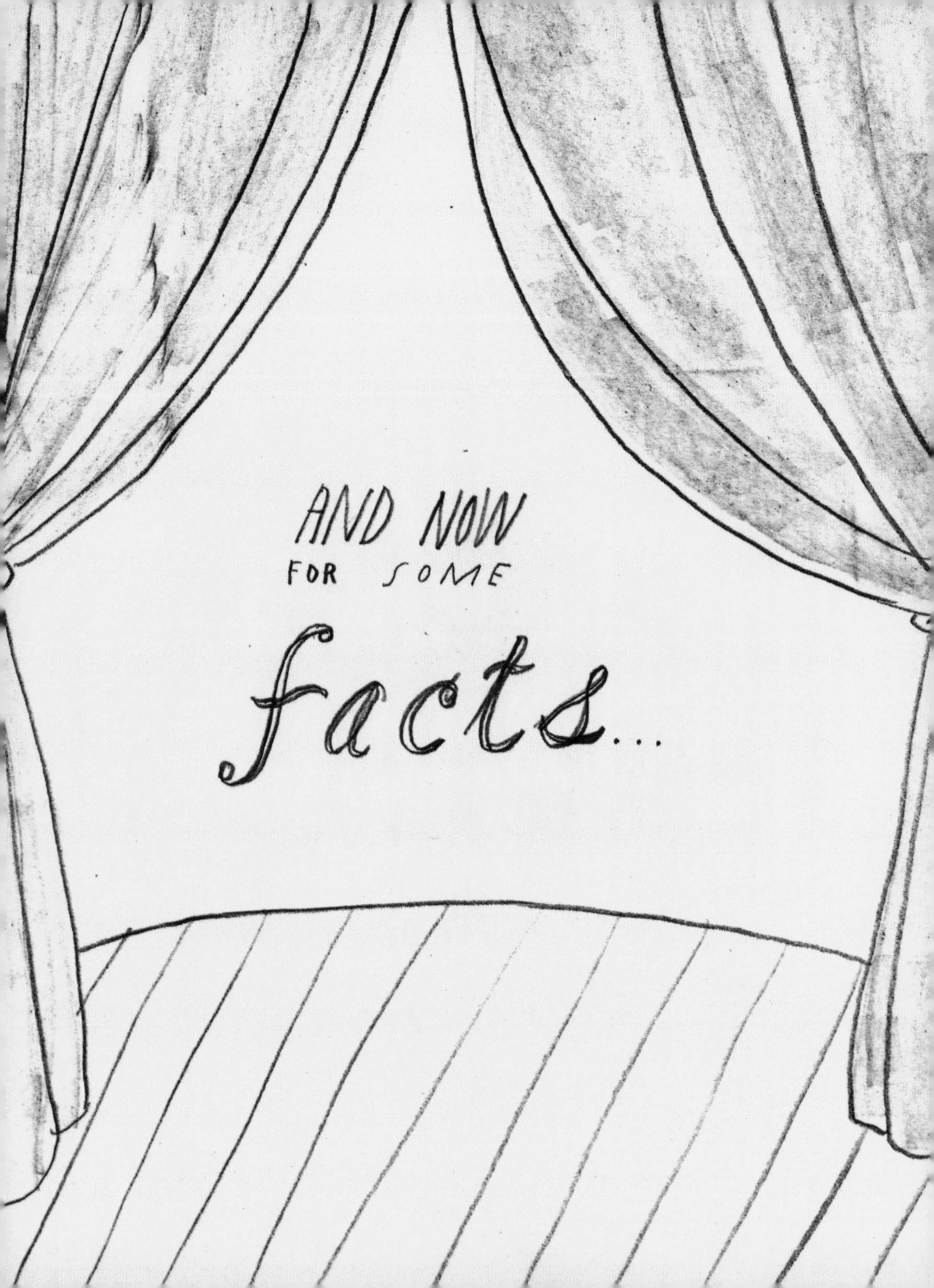
AND NOW
FOR SOME
facts...

AS WE MENTIONED EARLIER,
THERE ARE 2 KINDS OF ABORTION
PROCEDURES: "SURGICAL" AND "MEDICAL".
A SURGICAL ABORTION USES
SURGERY TO ABORT THE PREGNANCY
(AND HAPPENS IN A CLINIC).
A MEDICAL ABORTION INVOLVES
THE USE OF "ABORTIFACIENTS"
(MEDICATION).

* ALTHOUGH THIS INFORMATION MIGHT
BE HELPFUL AN' ALL... YOU MUST
STILL CALL A HEALTH OFFICIAL TO
ASK QUESTIONS! REMEMBER:
THIS IS A BOOK, NOT A DOCTOR!!

YOU HAVE THE OPTION OF HAVING A
MEDICAL ABORTION UP TO ABOUT 9
WEEKS (YOUR FIRST TRIMESTER) INTO YOUR
PREGNANCY. AFTER THAT... YOU MUST
HAVE A SURGICAL PROCEDURE (TOO RISKY
FOR A LOT O' REASONS!). THERE ARE
PROS + CONS TO EACH PROCEDURE,
SO IF IT IS STILL EARLY ENOUGH
TO CHOOSE, FIND OUT AS MUCH AS
YOU CAN FROM YOUR DOCTOR AND THEN
CHOOSE WHAT IS RIGHT FOR YOU.

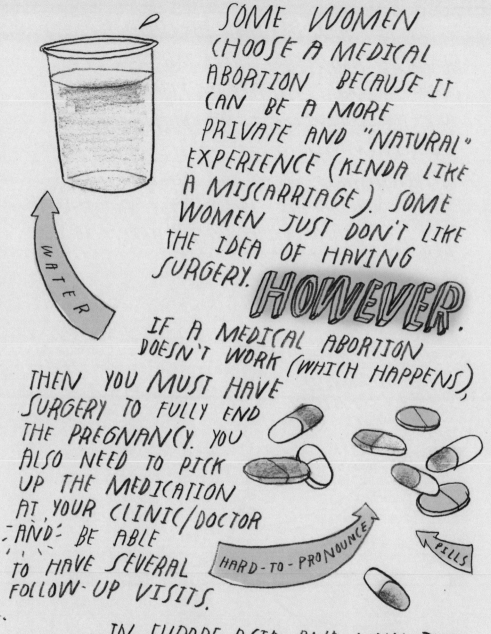

SOME WOMEN CHOOSE A MEDICAL ABORTION BECAUSE IT CAN BE A MORE PRIVATE AND "NATURAL" EXPERIENCE (KINDA LIKE A MISCARRIAGE). SOME WOMEN JUST DON'T LIKE THE IDEA OF HAVING SURGERY. **HOWEVER**.

WATER

IF A MEDICAL ABORTION DOESN'T WORK (WHICH HAPPENS), THEN YOU MUST HAVE SURGERY TO FULLY END THE PREGNANCY. YOU ALSO NEED TO PICK UP THE MEDICATION AT YOUR CLINIC/DOCTOR AND BE ABLE TO HAVE SEVERAL FOLLOW-UP VISITS.

HARD-TO-PRONOUNCE

PILLS

IN EUROPE, ASIA, AND NOW THE U.S.A... THE MOST COMMONLY USED EARLY TRIMESTER MEDICATION FOR MEDICAL ABORTIONS IS A COMBINATION OF **MIFEPRISTONE** & **MISOPROSTOL**.

IF YOU DECIDE TO HAVE A MEDICAL ABORTION, THEN YOU WILL HAVE TO MAKE AN APPOINTMENT TO GET THE MEDICATION. YOU WILL HAVE AN EXAM, INCLUDING AN ULTRASOUND, TO DETERMINE HOW FAR ALONG YOU ARE. THEN YOUR DOCTOR WILL GIVE YOU THE PILLS, EXPLAIN WHAT WILL HAPPEN TO YOU, AND SEND YOU HOME.

MIFEPRISTONE "BLOCKS THE ACTION OF THE HORMONE(S) NEEDED TO SUSTAIN A PREGNANCY". IT'S CONSIDERED SAFE AND EFFECTIVE.[1]
...AND FIRST DEVELOPED IN FRANCE!
BERET

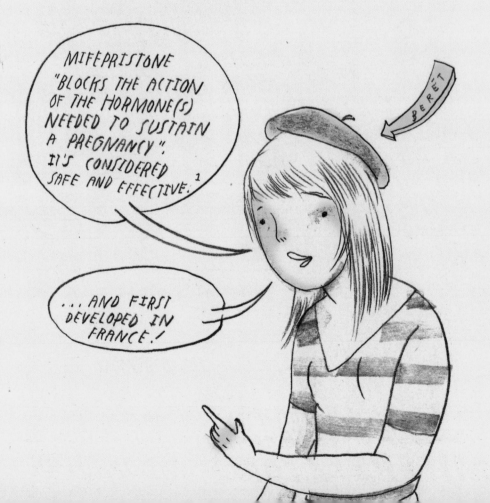

YOUR DOCTOR WILL
TELL YOU ABOUT WHAT
TO EXPECT. HE OR SHE
WILL WARN YOU THAT
THE MIFEPRISTONE CAN
CAUSE SOME PAINFUL
STUFF, LIKE CRAMPING.

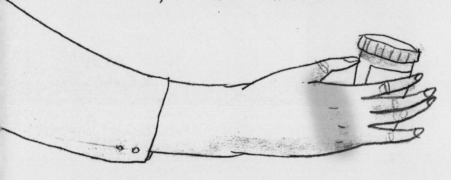

BUT DON'T BE AFRAID
TO ASK AS MANY
QUESTIONS AS YOU'D LIKE!
AFTER ALL: THAT'S WHAT THEY'RE
THERE FOR. NO QUESTION IS
TOO WEIRD.

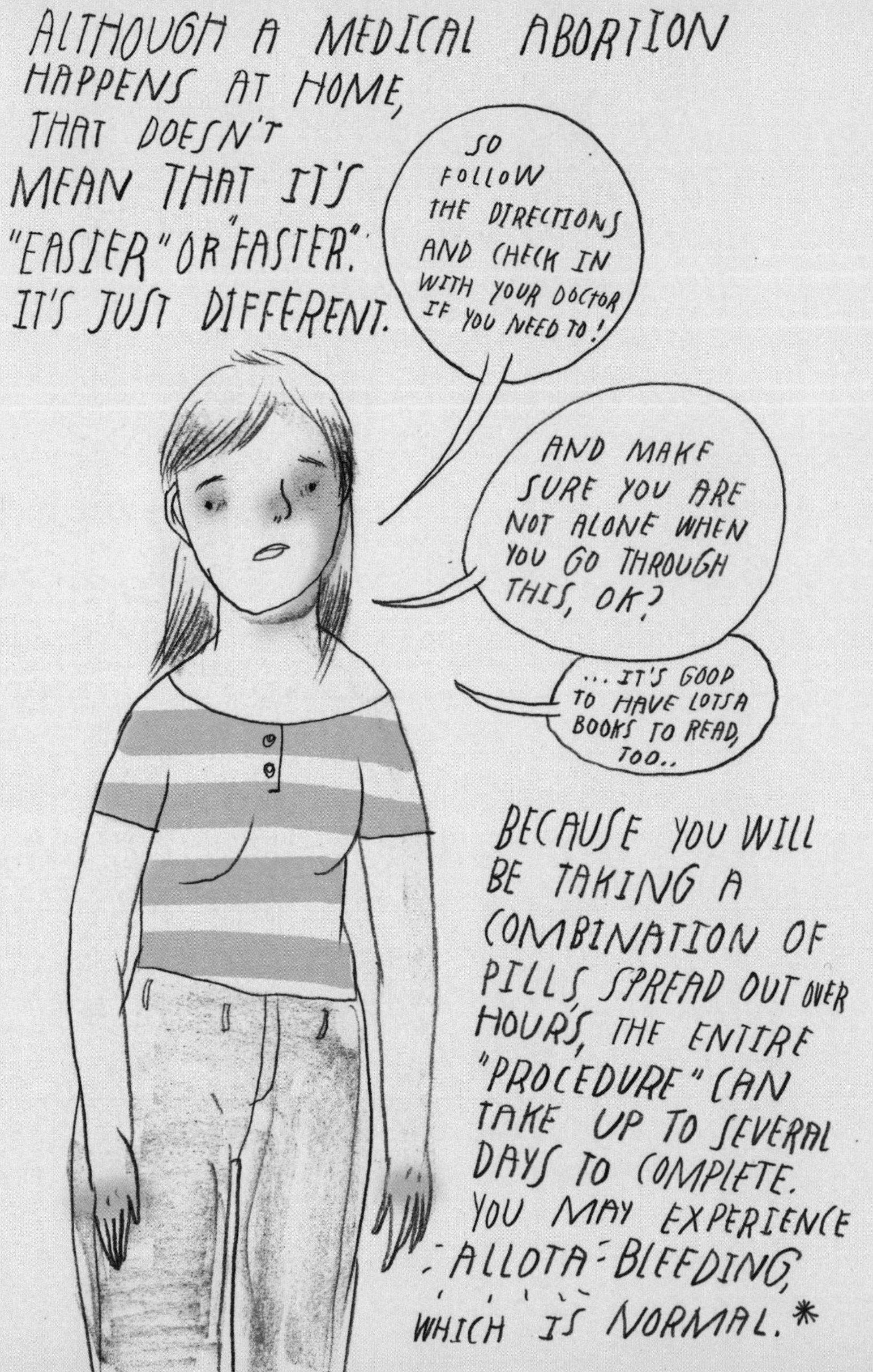
ALTHOUGH A MEDICAL ABORTION HAPPENS AT HOME, THAT DOESN'T MEAN THAT IT'S "EASIER" OR "FASTER". IT'S JUST DIFFERENT.
SO FOLLOW THE DIRECTIONS AND CHECK IN WITH YOUR DOCTOR IF YOU NEED TO!
AND MAKE SURE YOU ARE NOT ALONE WHEN YOU GO THROUGH THIS, OK?
...IT'S GOOD TO HAVE LOTSA BOOKS TO READ, TOO..
BECAUSE YOU WILL BE TAKING A COMBINATION OF PILLS SPREAD OUT OVER HOURS, THE ENTIRE "PROCEDURE" CAN TAKE UP TO SEVERAL DAYS TO COMPLETE. YOU MAY EXPERIENCE ALLOTA BLEEDING, WHICH IS NORMAL.*

* AND **ONE MORE** TIME (JUST FOR GOOD MEASURE), ALWAYS REFER TO A <u>DOCTOR</u> TO ANSWER YOUR QUESTIONS... NOT THE INTERNET, YOUR FRIENDS, OR EVEN THIS BOOK !! GOT THAT?

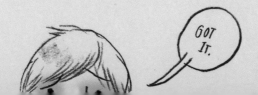

A SURGICAL

ABORTION IS DONE IN A CLINIC, HOSPITAL, OR DOCTOR'S OFFICE. IT IS A SURGERY (HENCE THE TERM), AND THE ENTIRE PROCEDURE IS DONE IN THE SAME DAY.

WHILE THE ACTUAL SURGERY TAKES A VERY SHORT AMOUNT OF TIME, SOMETIMES THERE IS A LOT OF WAITING AROUND IN WAITING ROOMS. BE PREPARED TO WATCH A LOT OF REALITY T.V.!

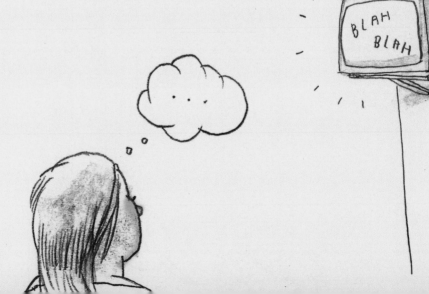

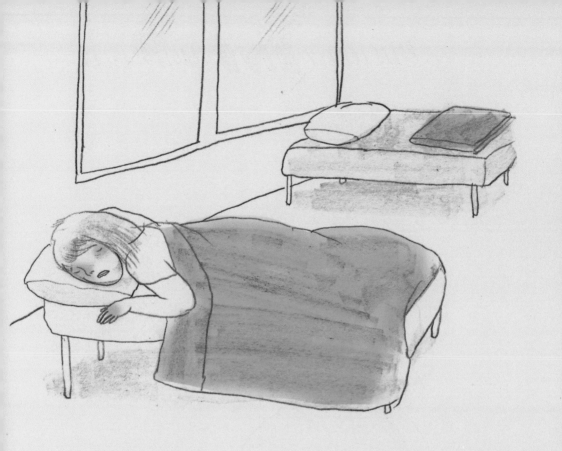

YOU WILL HAVE LOCAL ANESTHESIA.
THERE ARE PLACES FOR YOU TO SLEEP
IN THE RECOVERY ROOM, UNTIL YOU FEEL
BETTER ENOUGH TO GO HOME. BUT NO
MATTER WHAT: _ALWAYS_ HAVE A
FRIEND, PARTNER, FAMILY MEMBER, SOMEONE
BE THERE WHEN YOU GET OUT OF RECOVERY!!
YOU MAY FEEL PRETTY *WONKY...*

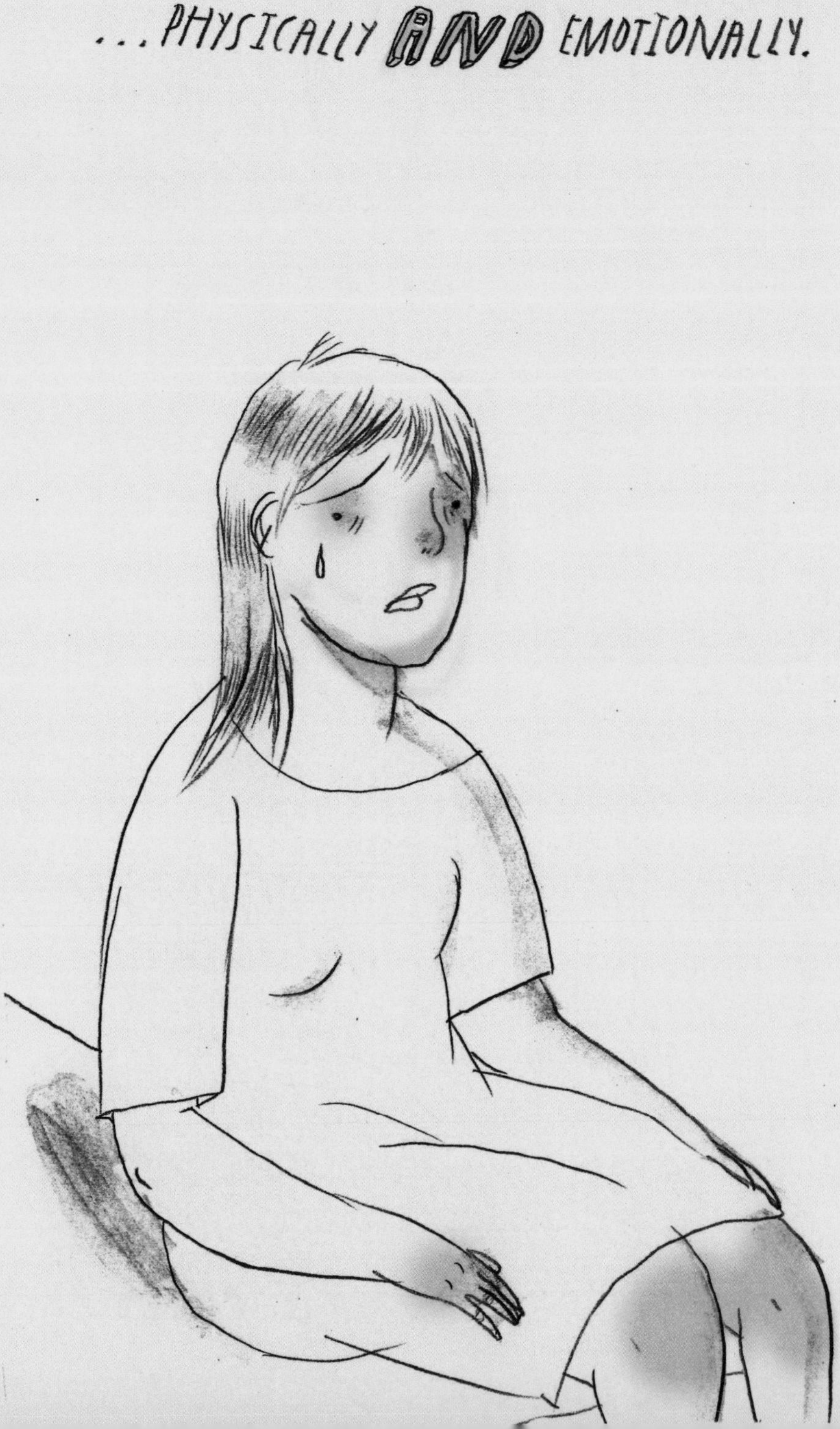
...PHYSICALLY AND EMOTIONALLY.

NOW.
BACK TO MARY
AND
LISA.

LISA THOUGHT ABOUT IT, AND TALKED TO HER SISTER ABOUT WHICH PROCEDURE TO HAVE. SHE HAD NO PROBLEM WITH HOSPITALS, AND WASN'T COMFORTABLE WITH THE IDEA OF DOING THE WHOLE THING AT HOME, SO SHE CHOSE THE SURGERY. HER SISTER TOLD HER THAT SHE WOULD BE THERE FOR HER NO MATTER WHAT SHE DECIDED TO DO.

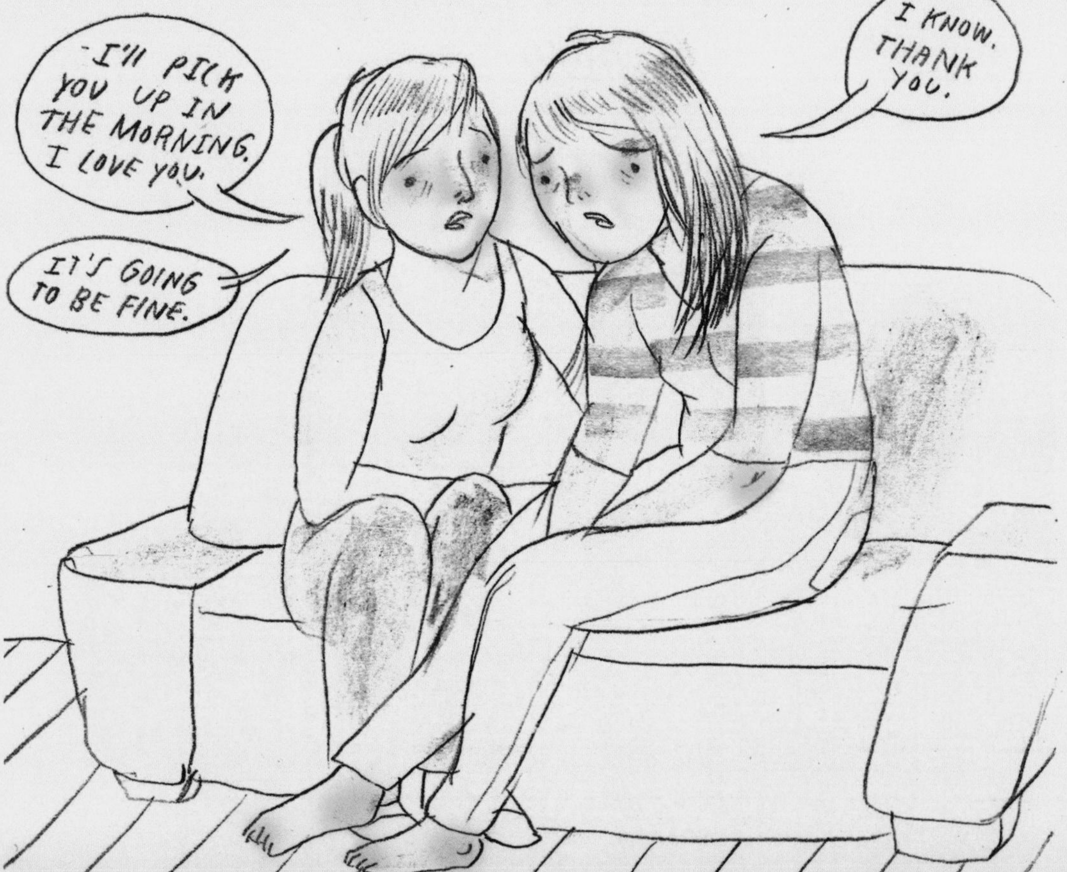

-I'LL PICK YOU UP IN THE MORNING. I LOVE YOU.
I KNOW. THANK YOU.
IT'S GOING TO BE FINE.

THERE WAS ANOTHER VERY IMPORTANT THING THAT NEEDED TO BE DONE. ALTHOUGH LISA WAS NOT WITH HER PARTNER ANYMORE, SHE CALLED AND TOLD HIM ABOUT WHAT SHE HAD FOUND OUT, AND WHAT SHE HAD DECIDED TO DO. HE WAS VERY SUPPORTIVE.

...IT'S YOURS. THIS IS HARD.
CAN I TAKE YOU? HOW CAN I HELP?
NO MY SISTER WILL.
CAN I PAY FOR IT?
OK.

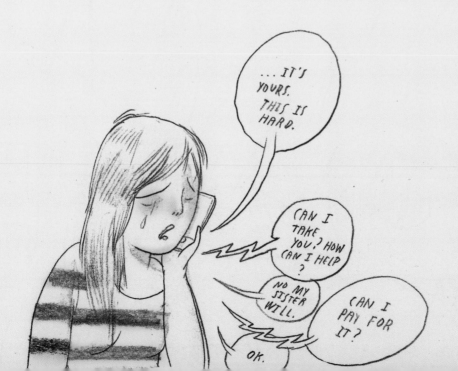

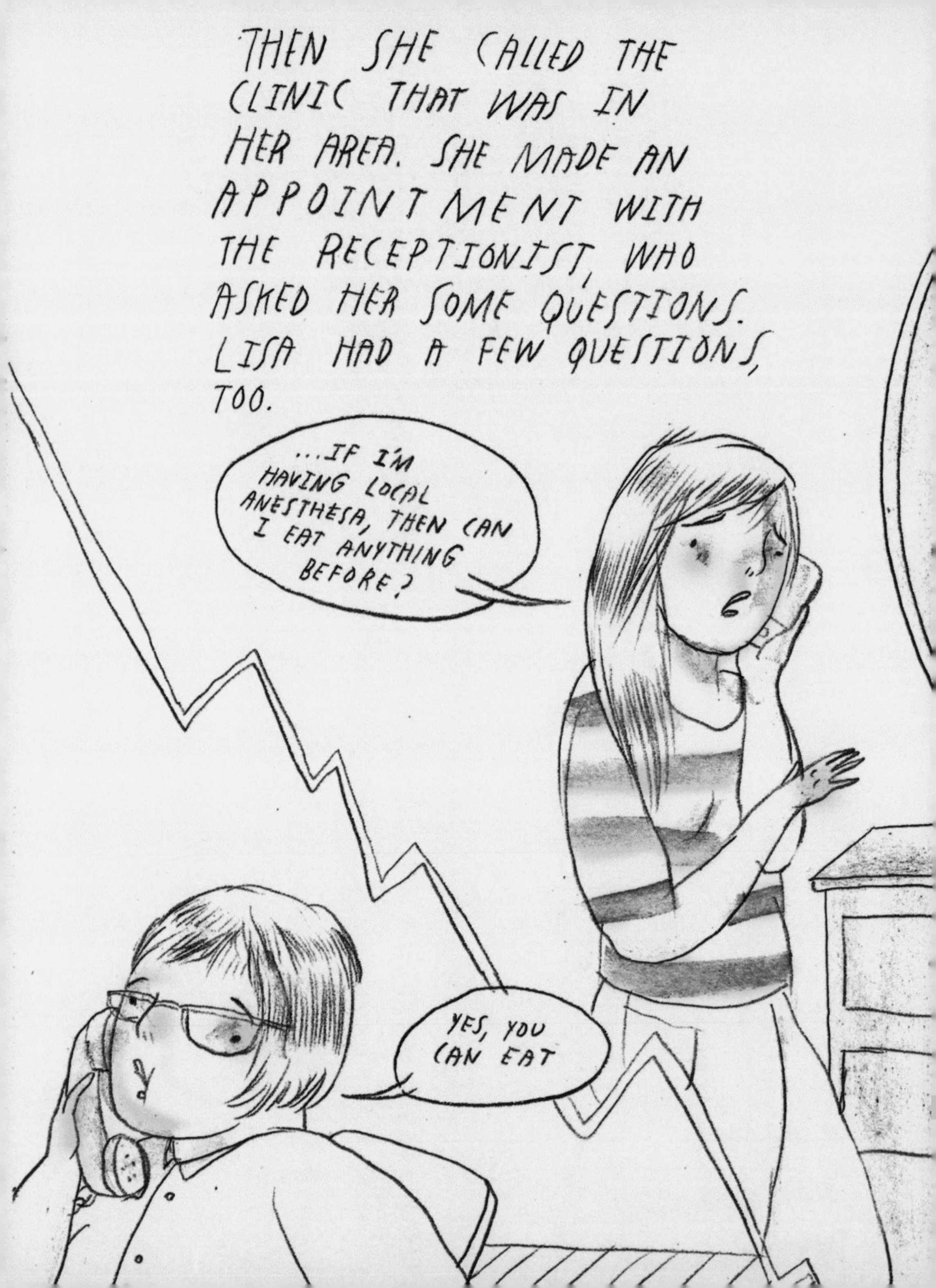
THEN SHE CALLED THE CLINIC THAT WAS IN HER AREA. SHE MADE AN APPOINTMENT WITH THE RECEPTIONIST, WHO ASKED HER SOME QUESTIONS. LISA HAD A FEW QUESTIONS, TOO.
...IF I'M HAVING LOCAL ANESTHESA, THEN CAN I EAT ANYTHING BEFORE?
YES, YOU CAN EAT

REMEMBER.

THIS IS <u>NOT</u> AN <u>EASY THING</u> TO GO THROUGH. DON'T BE AFRAID TO TALK TO SOMEONE (OR SOMEONES!) ABOUT WHAT YOU'RE FEELING.

NO MATTER HOW YOU GOT HERE, YOU WILL PROBABLY HAVE

A GAZZILION

THOUGHTS AND FEELINGS RUNNING THROUGH YOUR HEAD.

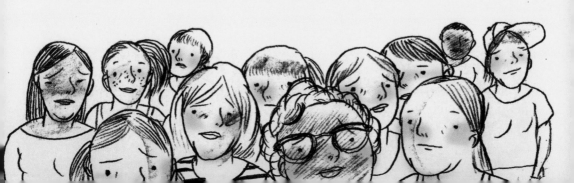

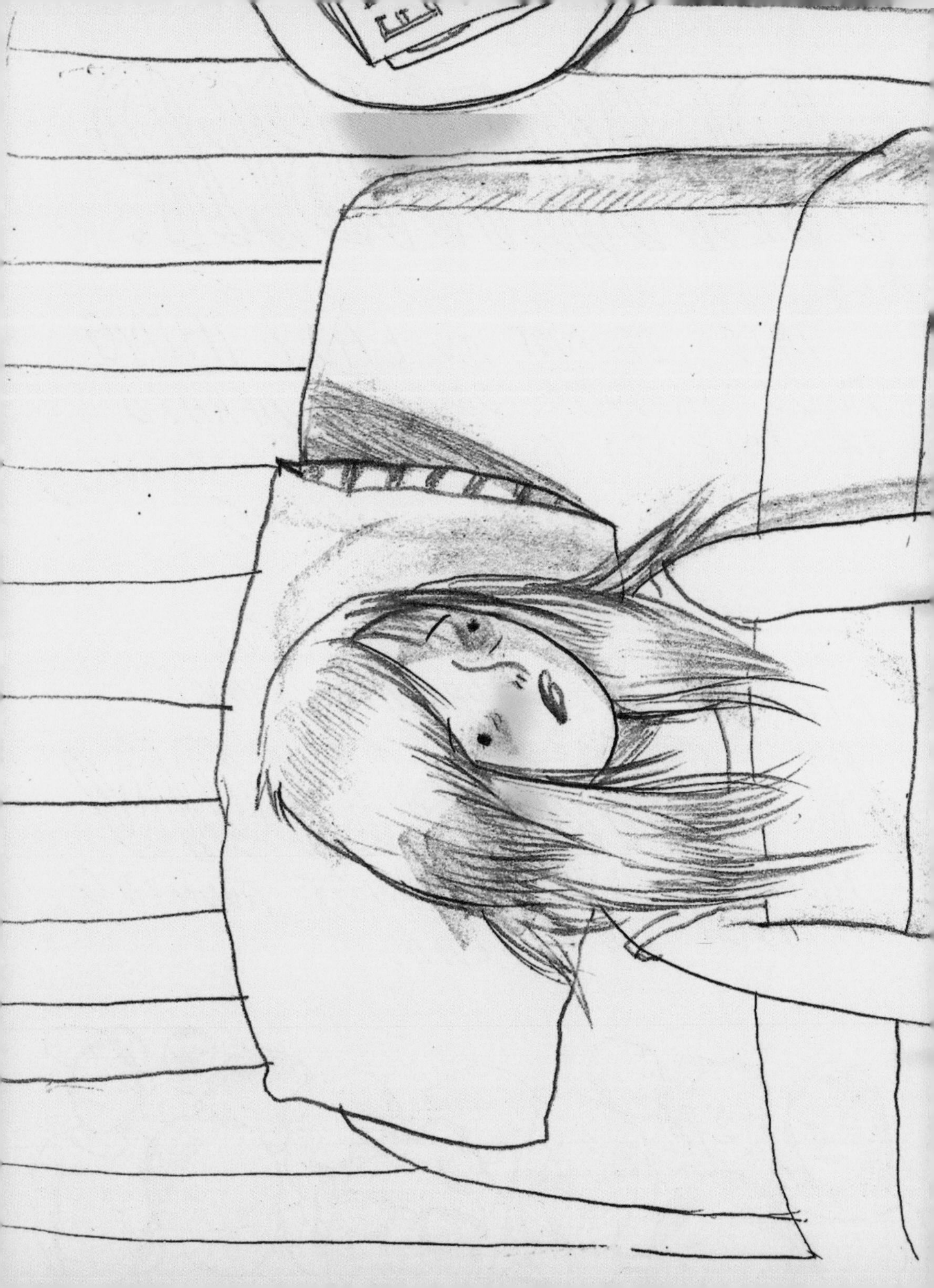

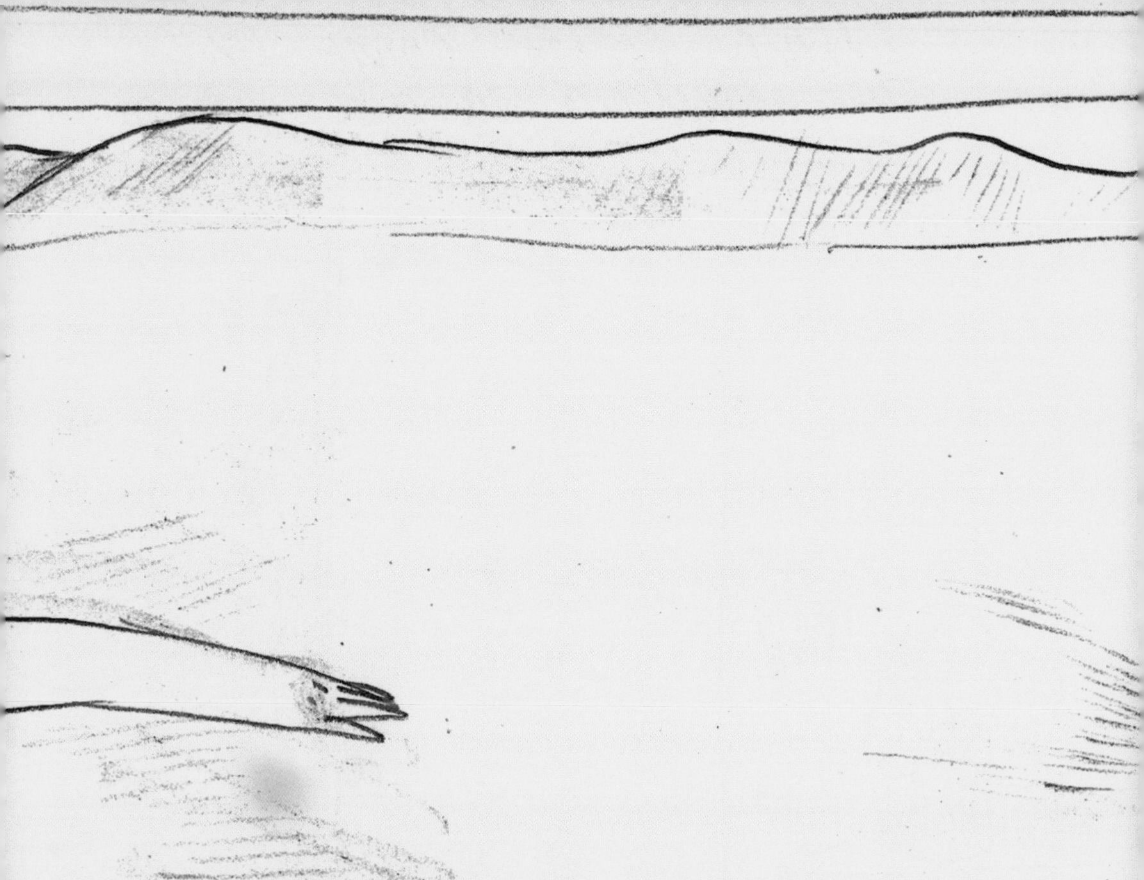

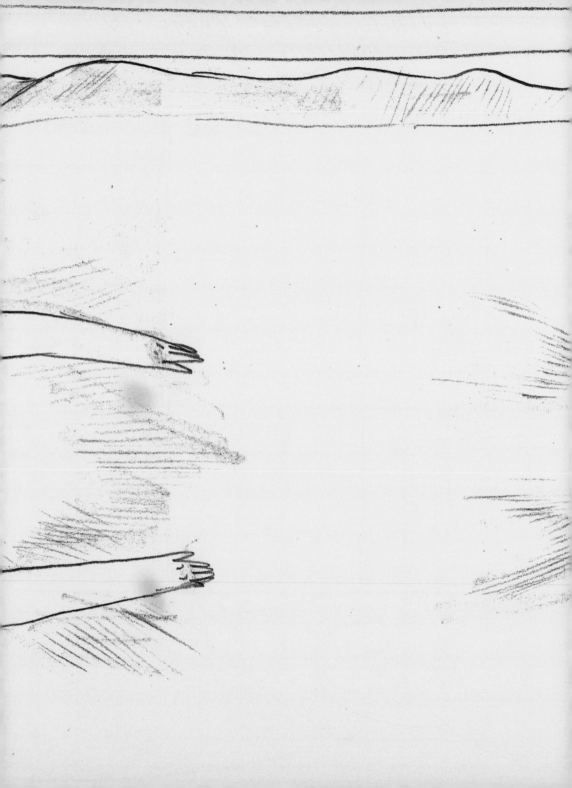

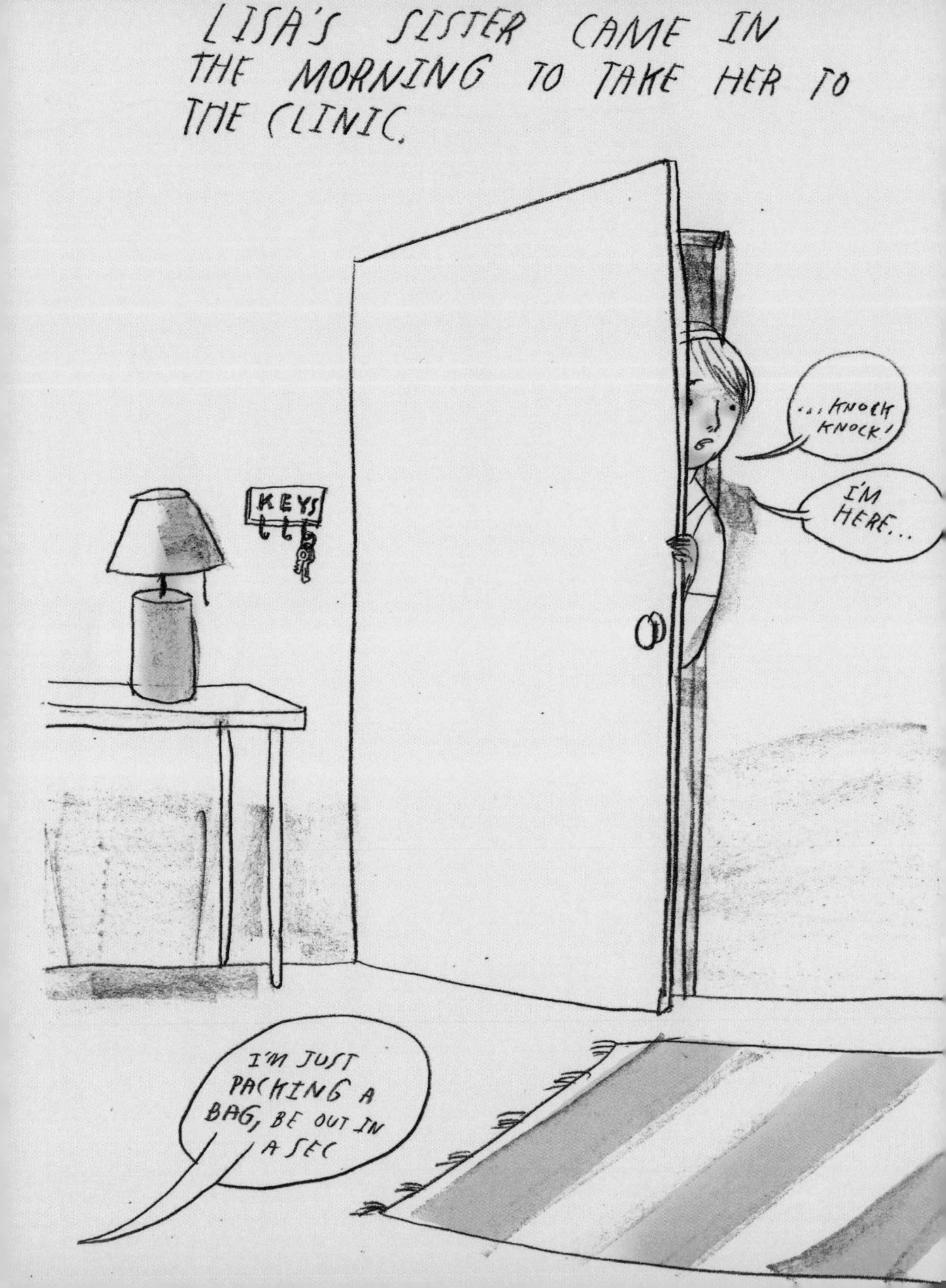
LISA'S SISTER CAME IN THE MORNING TO TAKE HER TO THE CLINIC.
...KNOCK KNOCK!
I'M HERE...
I'M JUST PACKING A BAG, BE OUT IN A SEC

WHEN YOU ARE ABOUT TO DO SOMETHING SCARY, IT'S FUNNY HOW DIFFERENT THE WORLD CAN SUDDENLY SEEM.

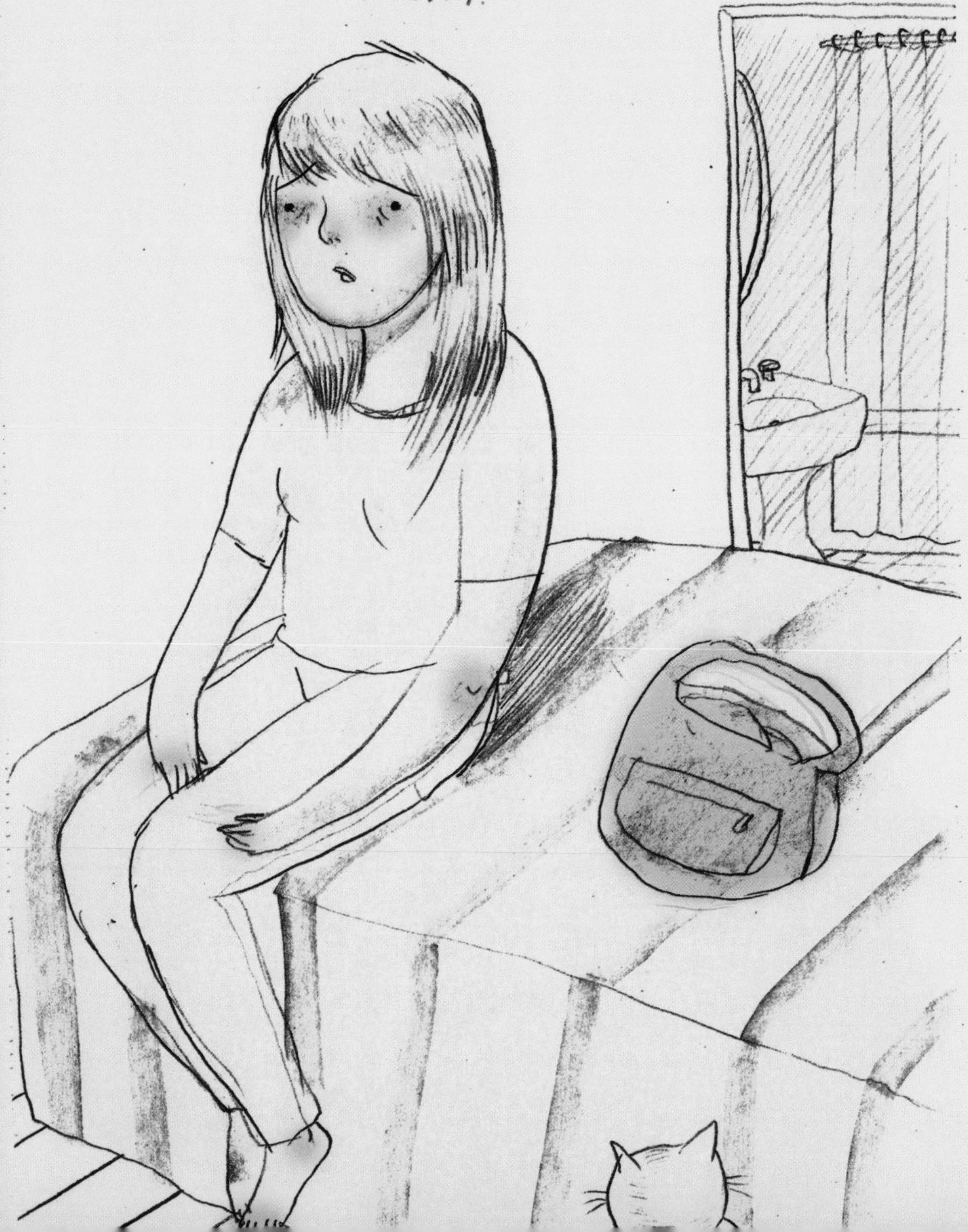

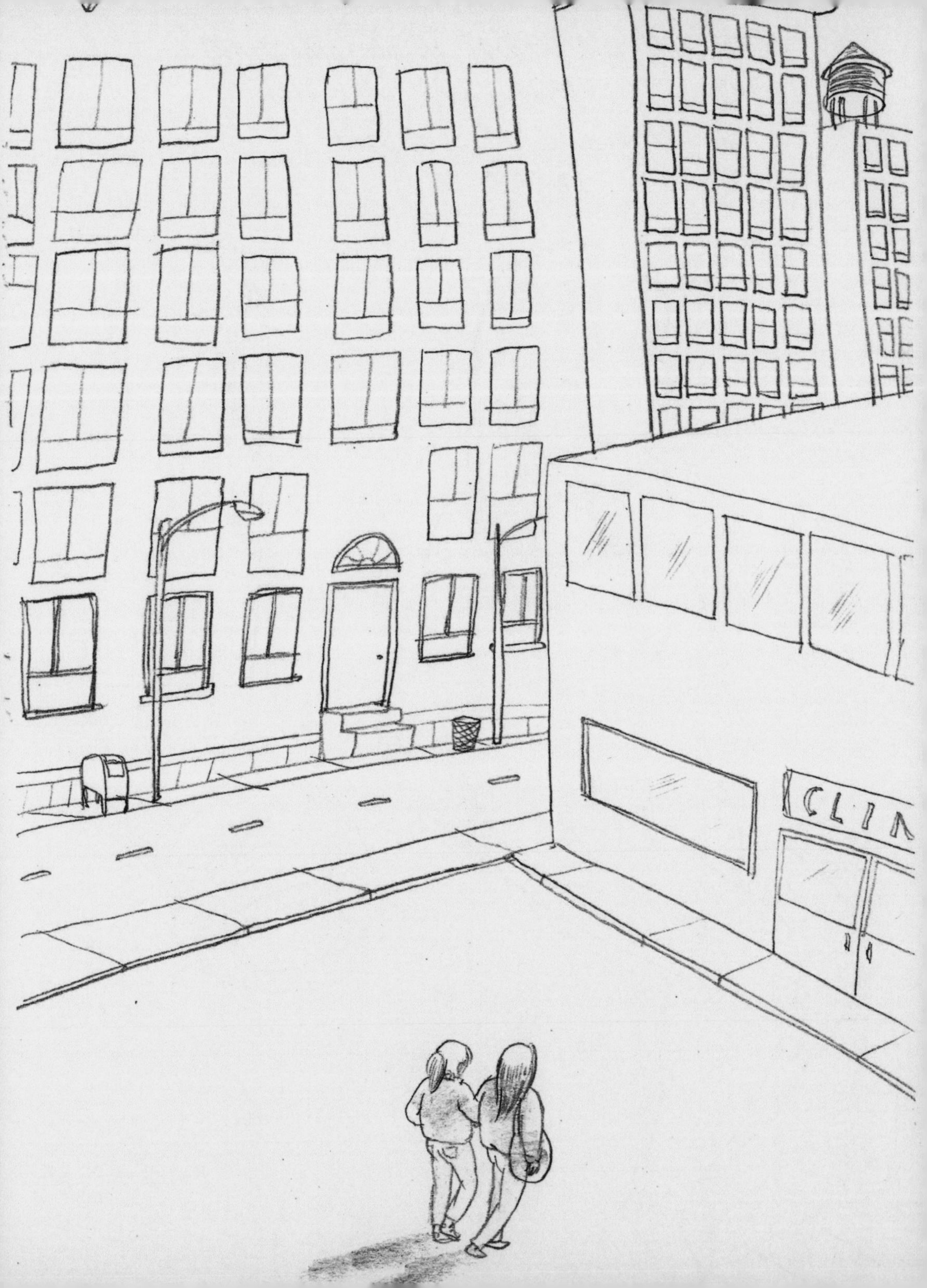
CLI

THE **CLINIC** WAS IN THE CITY, DOWN A BUSY STREET.

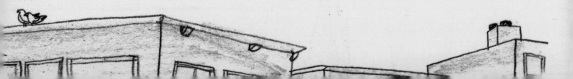

THERE WAS A SECURITY GUARD INSIDE. LISA HAD TO SIGN IN AND FILL OUT SOME INFORMATION.

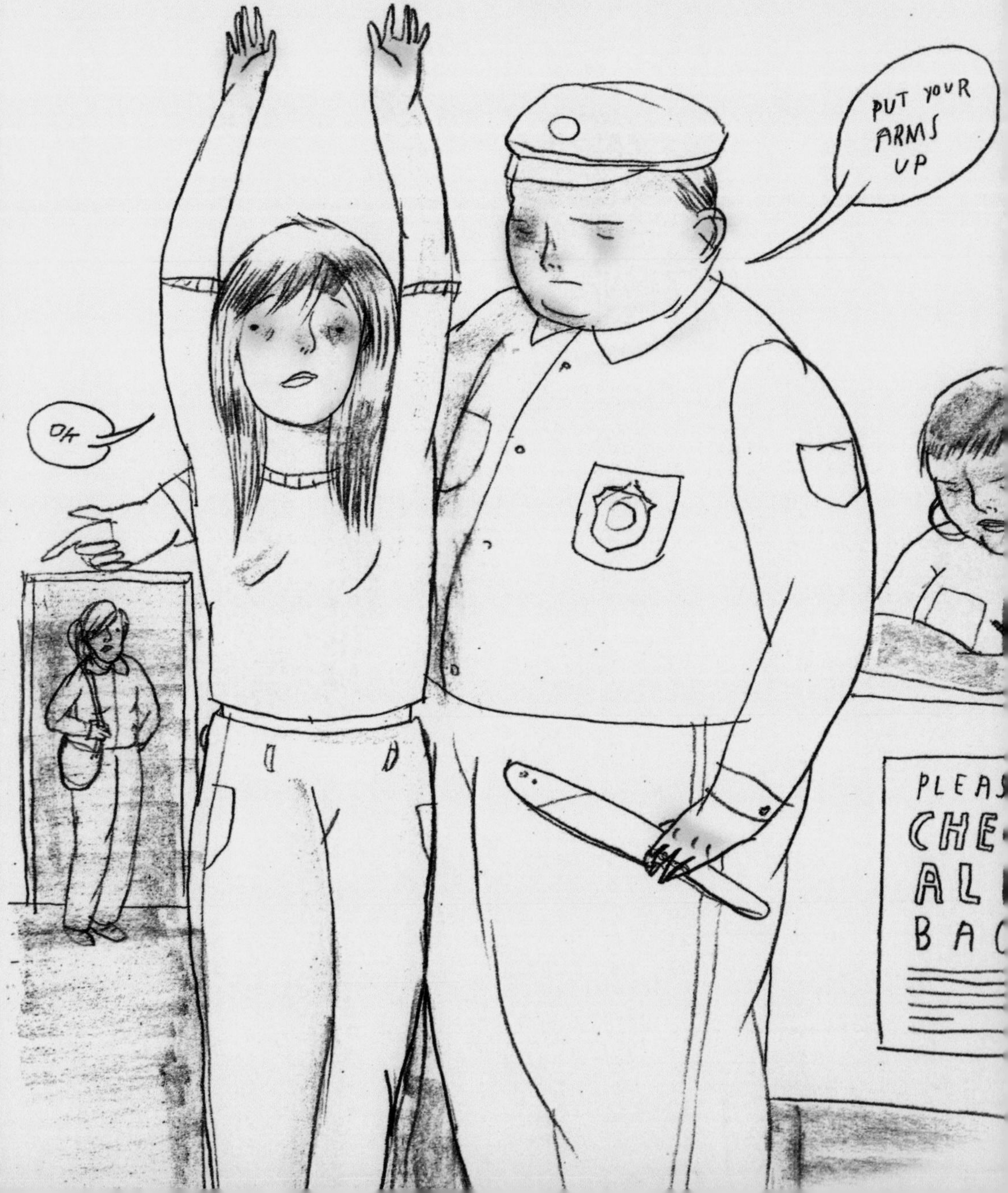
PUT YOUR ARMS UP
OK
PLEAS
CHE
AL
BAC

LISA'S SISTER WASN'T ALLOWED PAST A CERTAIN POINT, SO SHE STAYED DOWNSTAIRS TO WAIT.

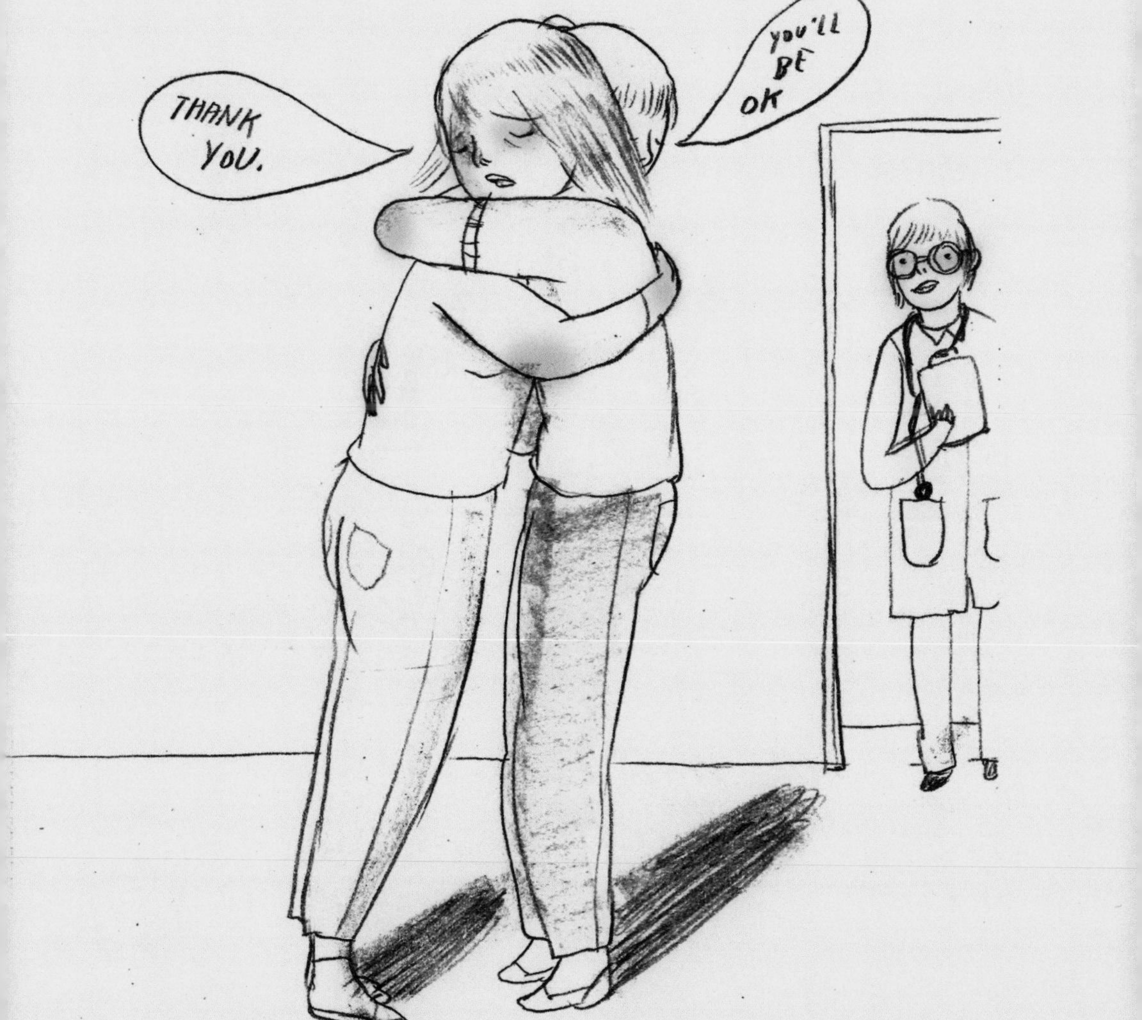
THANK YOU.
YOU'LL BE OK

ONLY PATIENTS ARE ALLOWED IN THE SURGERY AREA.

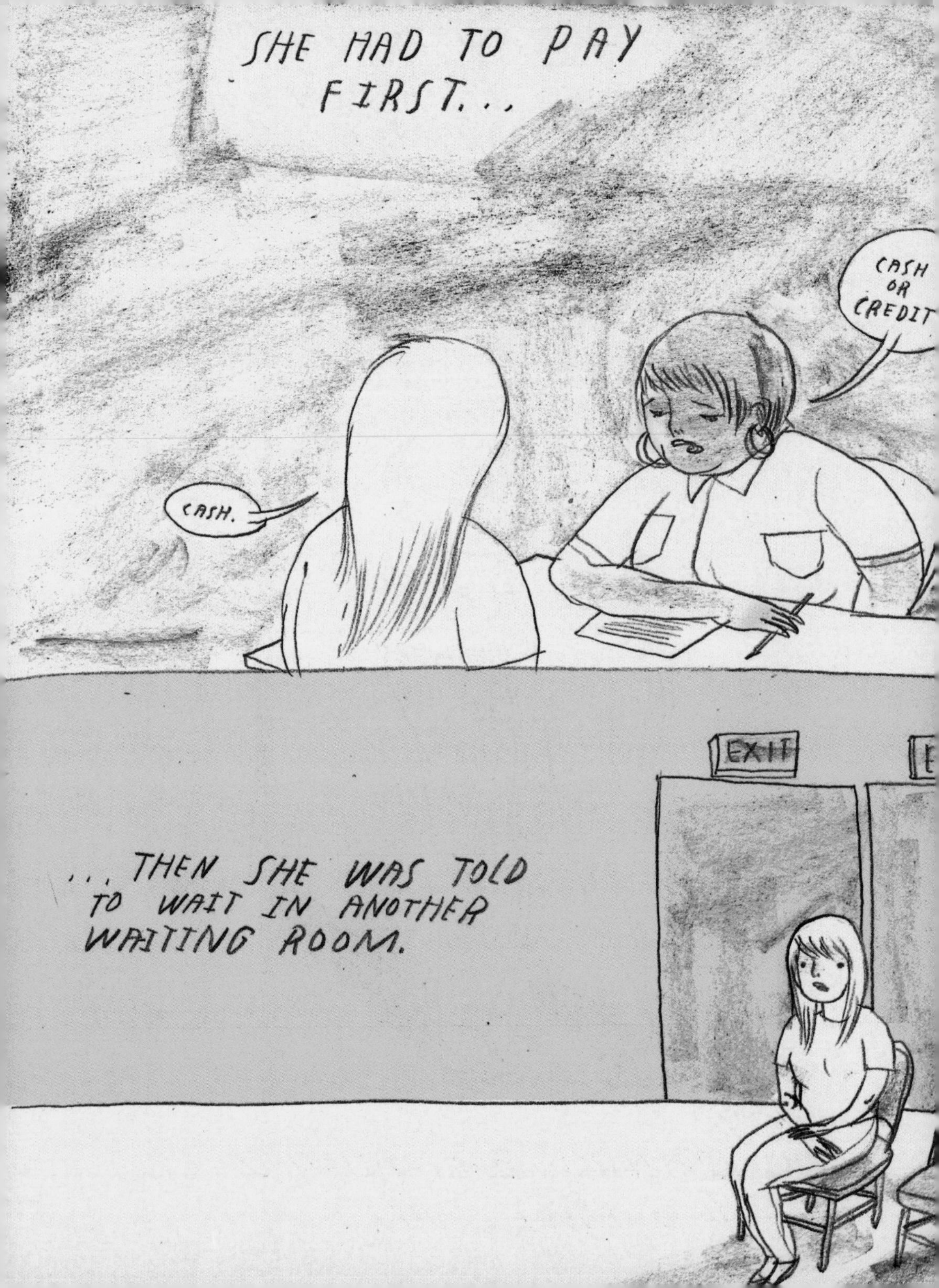
SHE HAD TO PAY FIRST...
CASH OR CREDIT
CASH.
EXIT
...THEN SHE WAS TOLD TO WAIT IN ANOTHER WAITING ROOM.

SHE WAITED FOR WHAT
SEEMED LIKE A LONG
TIME.

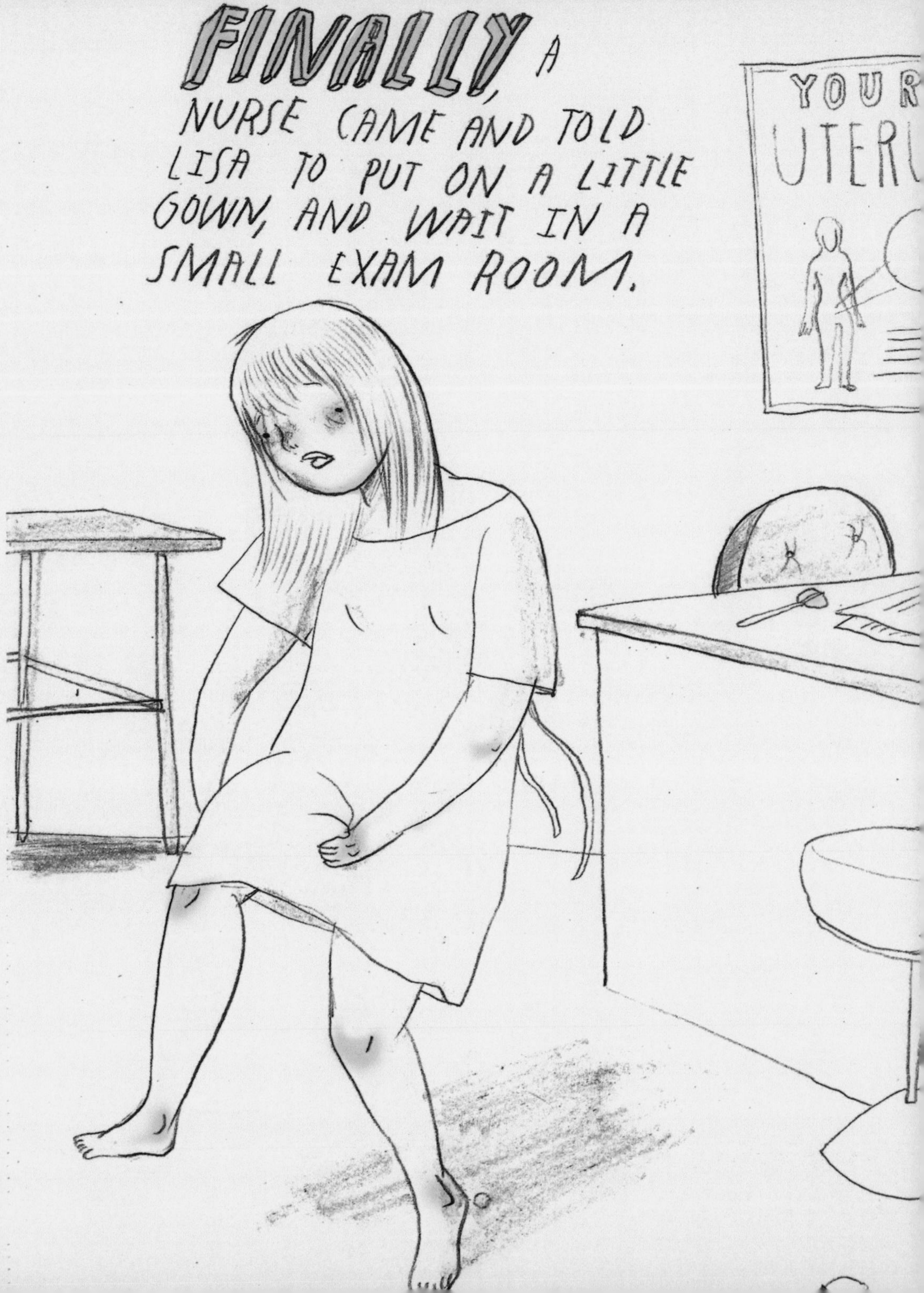
FINALLY, A NURSE CAME AND TOLD LISA TO PUT ON A LITTLE GOWN, AND WAIT IN A SMALL EXAM ROOM.
YOUR
UTER

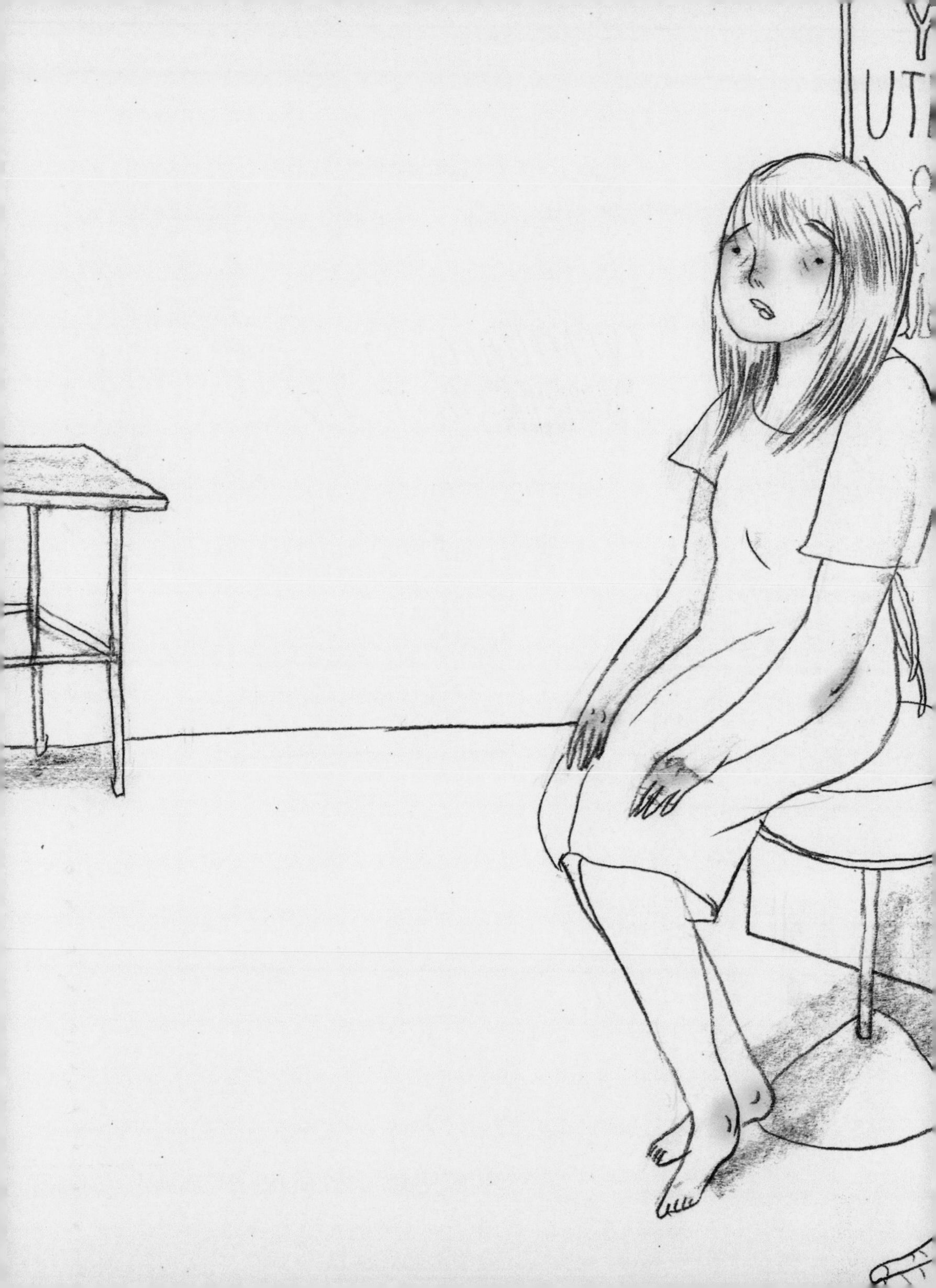

EVENTUALLY, A **NURSE** CAME IN.

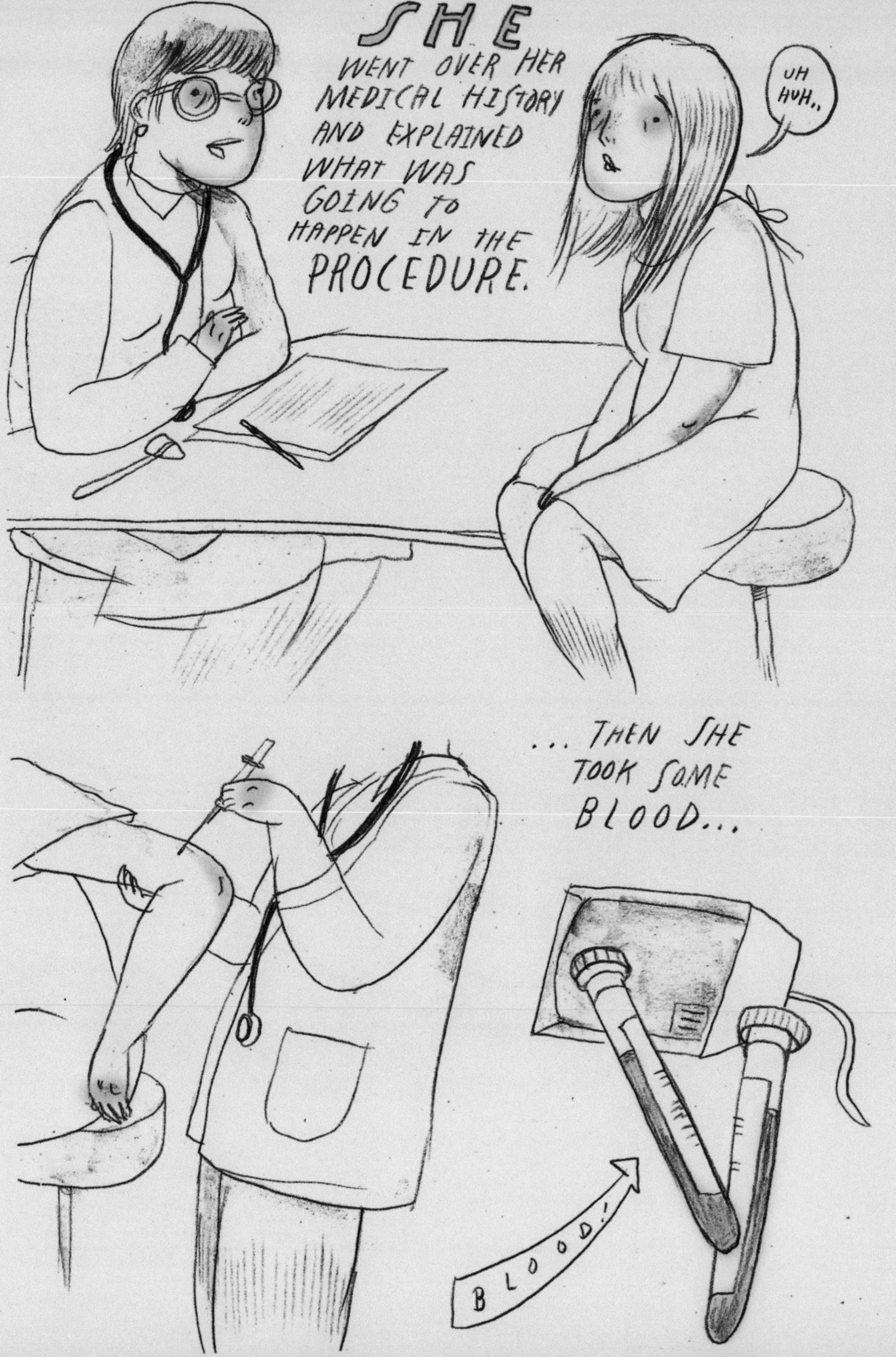
SHE WENT OVER HER MEDICAL HISTORY AND EXPLAINED WHAT WAS GOING TO HAPPEN IN THE PROCEDURE.
UH HUH..
...THEN SHE TOOK SOME BLOOD...
BLOOD!

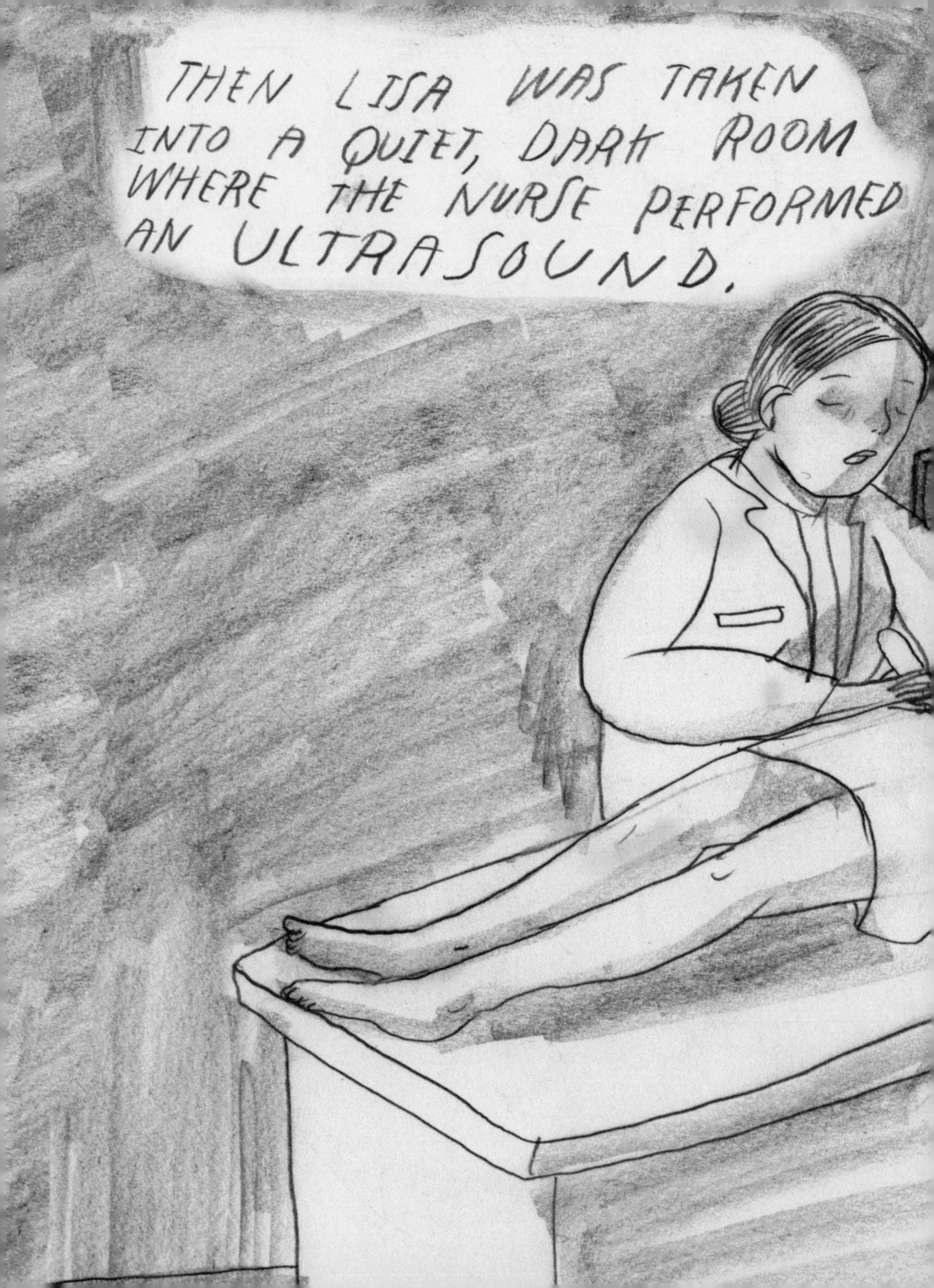
THEN LISA WAS TAKEN INTO A QUIET, DARK ROOM WHERE THE NURSE PERFORMED AN ULTRASOUND.

LISA DECIDED THAT
SHE DID NOT WANT
TO LOOK AT THE

SCREEN.

SOME GIRLS DO, AND
SOME GIRLS FIND THAT
THEY WOULD RATHER NOT
SEE A VISUAL OF WHAT'S
GOING ON IN THERE. EITHER
WAY, IT'S FINE!

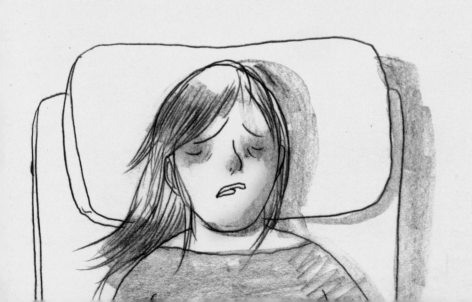

... THEN LISA WAS SENT TO WAIT IN
ANOTHER ROOM UNTIL IT WAS HER
TURN FOR SURGERY. THERE WAS A
LOT OF WAITING.

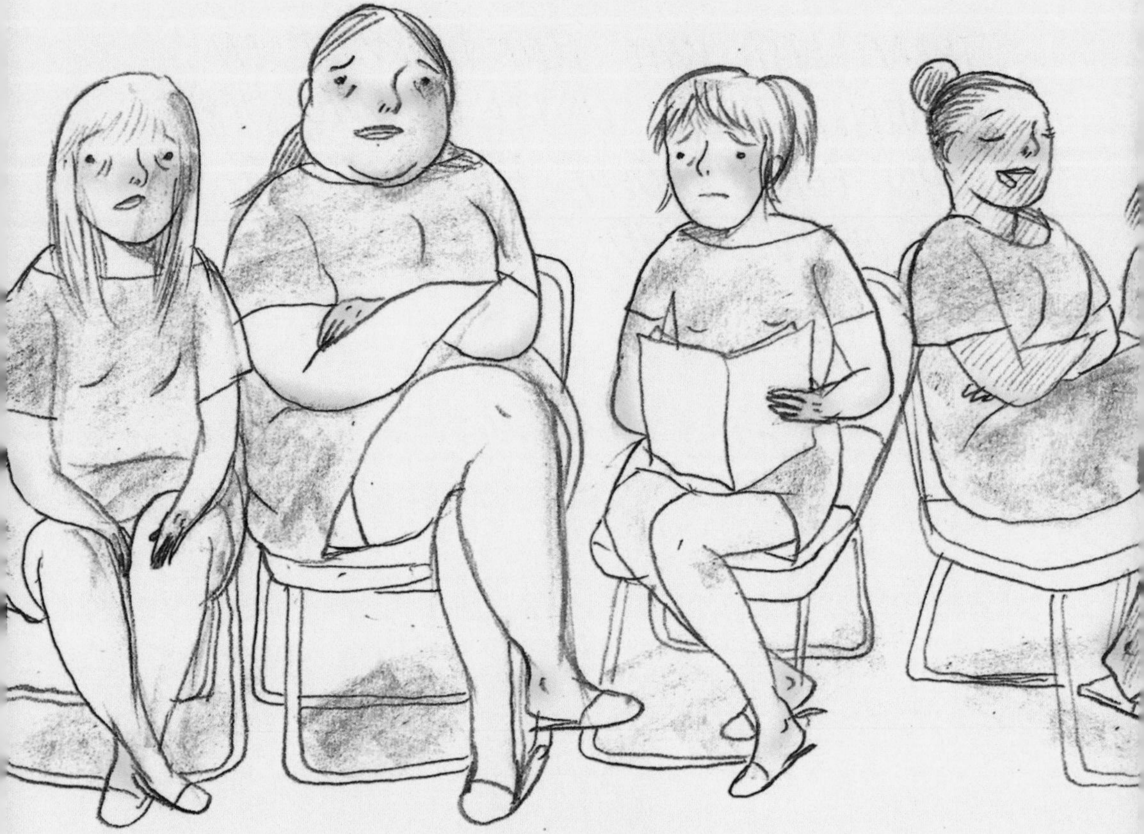

THERE WERE WOMEN OF ALL AGES, COLORS, BACKGROUNDS. SOME LOOKED SCARED, SOME WERE CHATTING WITH OTHER WOMEN. SOME WERE SILENT.

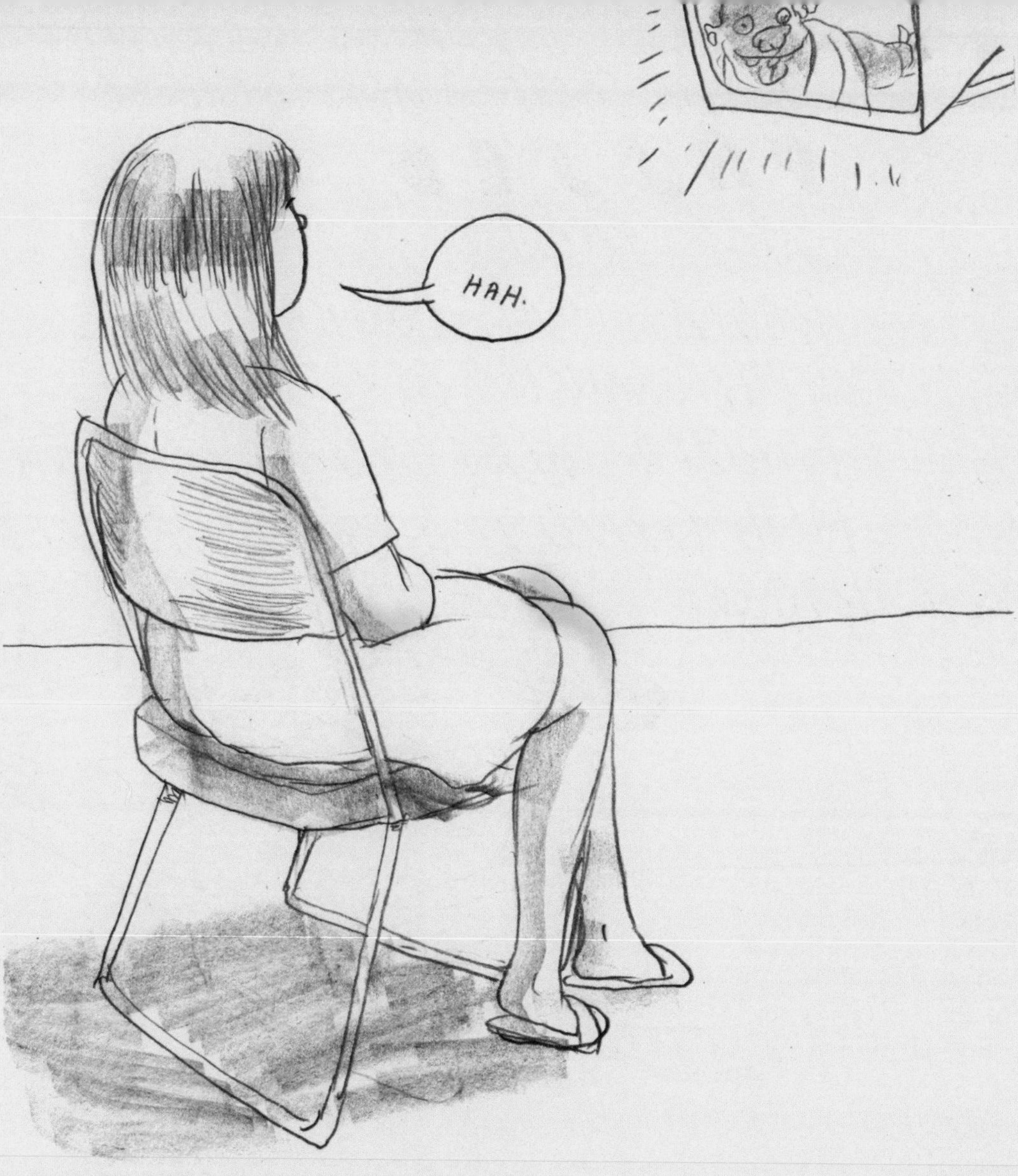
HAH.

SHE WATCHED "SHREK" (WHICH SHE HAD NEVER SEEN BEFORE). IT WAS PRETTY GOOD.

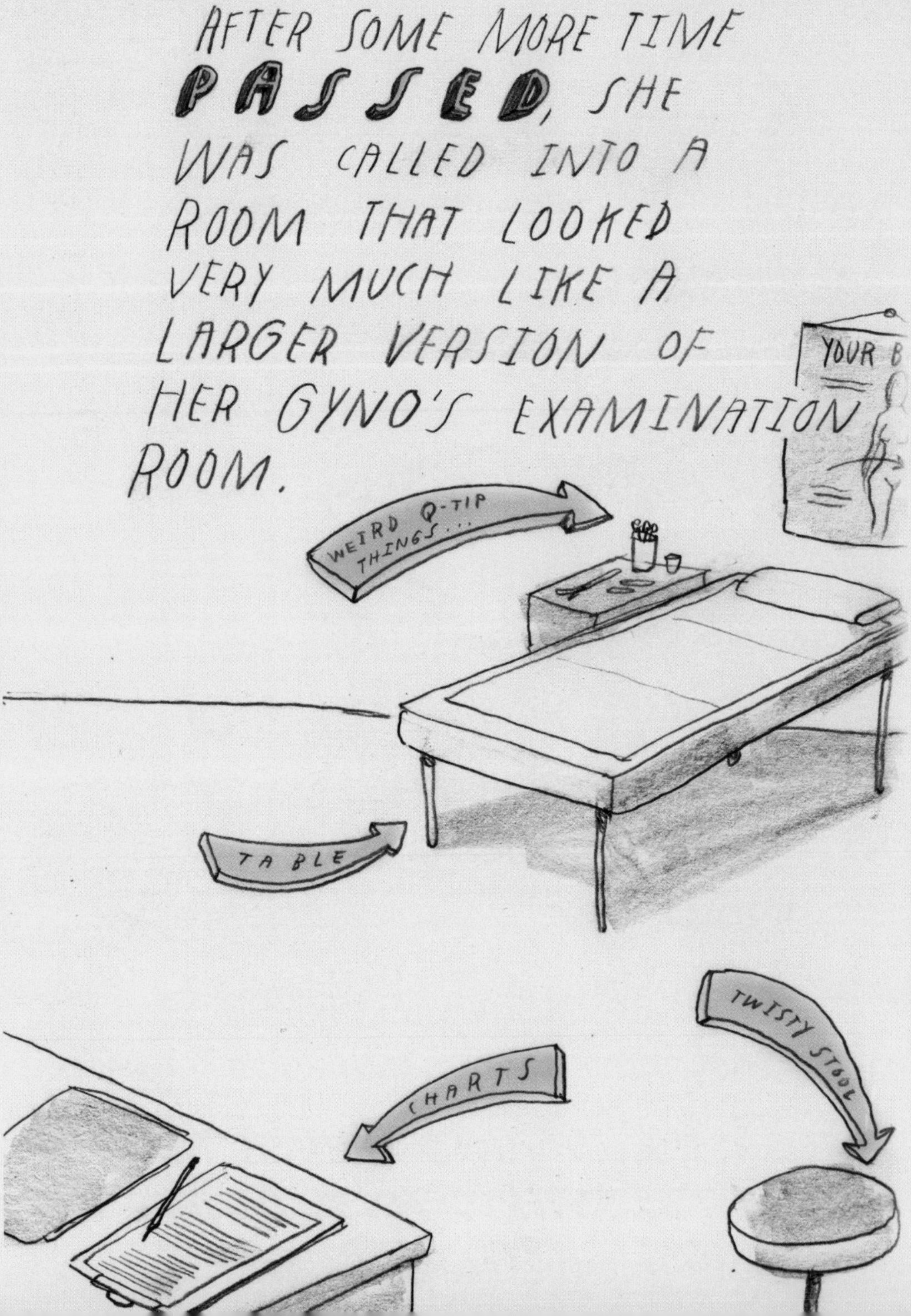
AFTER SOME MORE TIME PASSED, SHE WAS CALLED INTO A ROOM THAT LOOKED VERY MUCH LIKE A LARGER VERSION OF HER GYNO'S EXAMINATION ROOM.
WEIRD Q-TIP THINGS...
TABLE
TWISTY STOOL
CHARTS

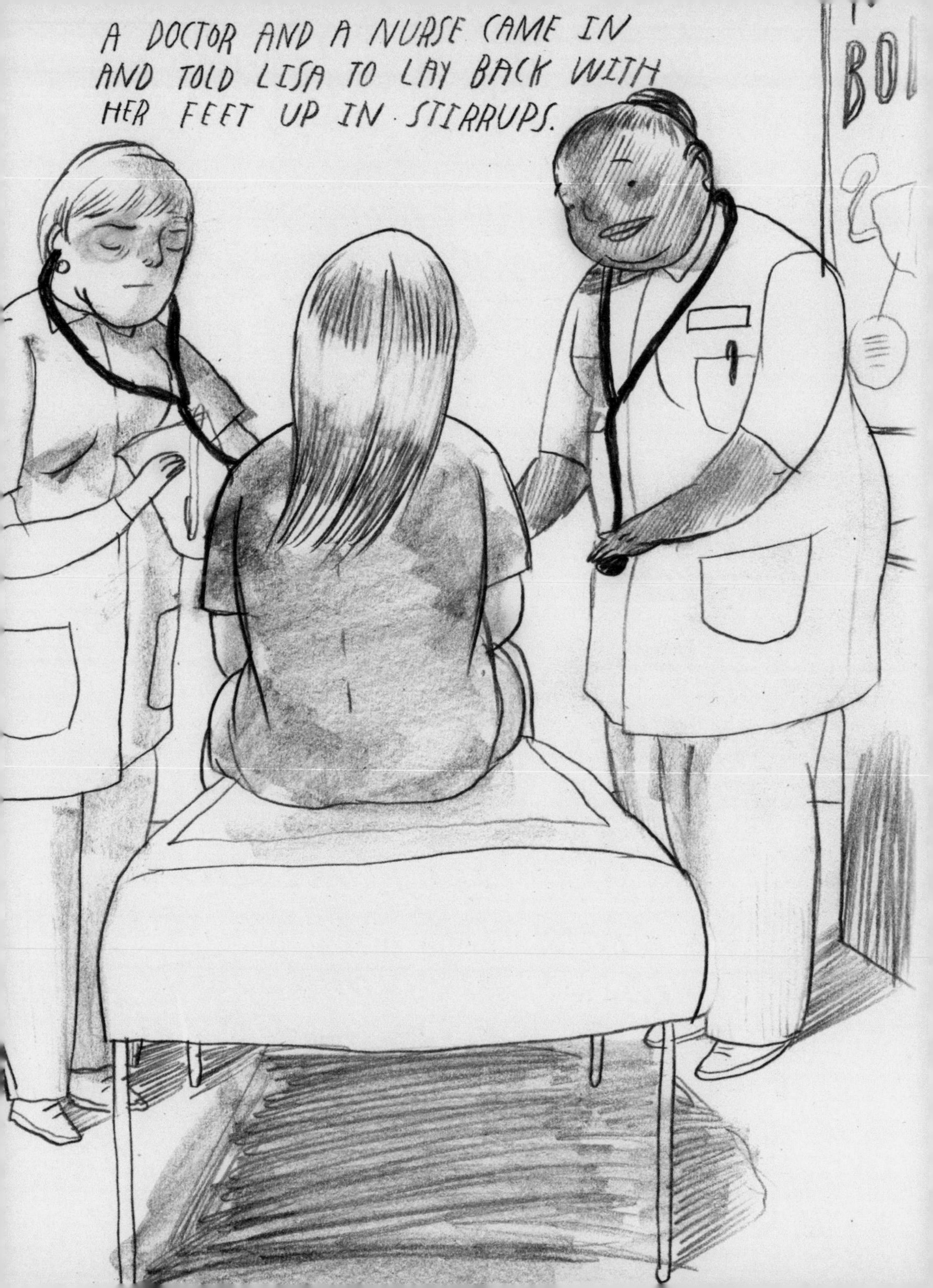
A DOCTOR AND A NURSE CAME IN AND TOLD LISA TO LAY BACK WITH HER FEET UP IN STIRRUPS.

BY THE WAY:

THIS KIND OF ABORTION IS CALLED: **ASPIRATION,**

WHICH MEANS AN INSTRUMENT IS INSERTED INTO THE UTERUS TO SUCTION OUT THE FETUS AND PLACENTA, AFTER CAREFULLY DIALATING THE CERVIX.

THIS IS WHY AN ANESTHETIC IS GIVEN. EVEN IF YOU ARE **AWAKE,** YOU MAY FEEL SOME PRESSURE INSIDE, SOME CRAMPING, OR YOU MAY FEEL FAINT AT TIMES.

DON'T WORRY.

THIS IS NORMAL!!

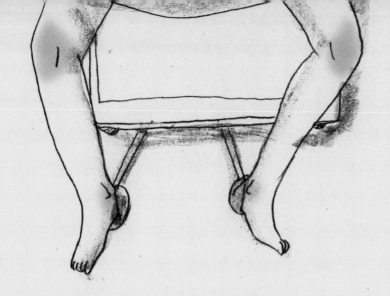

LISA FELT LIKE SHE
WAS AT A VISIT TO THE
GYNECOLOGIST AT FIRST.
EVERYTHING HAPPENED PRETTY
FAST. BUT THINGS SEEMED
DIFFERENT WHEN THE NURSE
GAVE HER THE LOCAL ANESTHESA.
SUDDENLY SHE COULD NOT
FEEL ANYTHING BETWEEN HER
LEGS. SHE LOOKED AT THE CEILING
AND WAITED FOR THE PROCEDURE
TO START.

THERE WAS A
LOT OF CRAMPING..
KIND OF LIKE GETTING A
PAP SMEAR
BUT AT TIMES, MORE INTENSE.
SHE TRIED TO BE VERY
BRAVE EVERY TIME IT HURT.
THE PROCEDURE TAKES A
VERY SHORT AMOUNT OF
TIME.

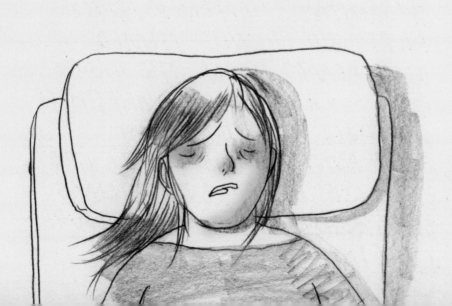

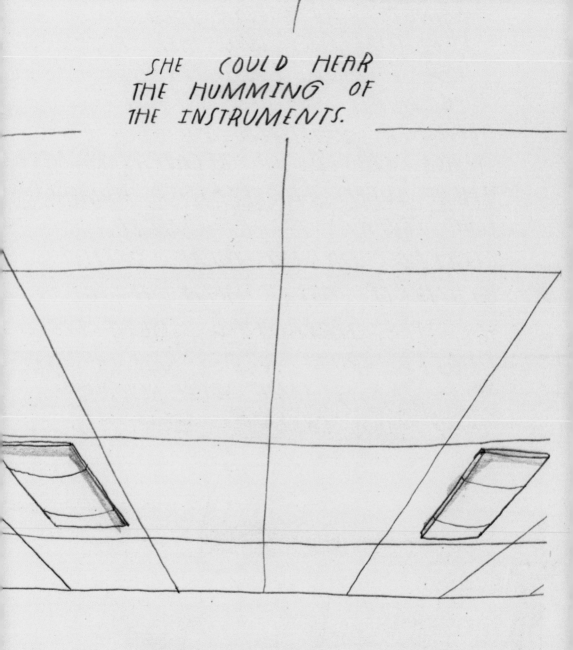

SHE COULD HEAR
THE HUMMING OF
THE INSTRUMENTS.

EXIT

AFTER ABOUT FIFTEEN MINUTES, THE DOCTOR TOLD HER THAT SHE WAS "ALL SET," AND HELPED LISA SIT UP. THE NURSE WALKED HER TO ANOTHER WAITING ROOM-LIKE PLACE CALLED THE "RECOVERY ROOM". THERE WERE BIG LEATHER ARMCHAIRS THAT SEVERAL GIRLS WERE CURLED UP IN, SOME WITH BLANKETS OVER THEM. A LOT OF THE GIRLS HAD THEIR EYES CLOSED, BUT WERE NOT SLEEPING. SOME WERE READING, SOME WERE CRYING.

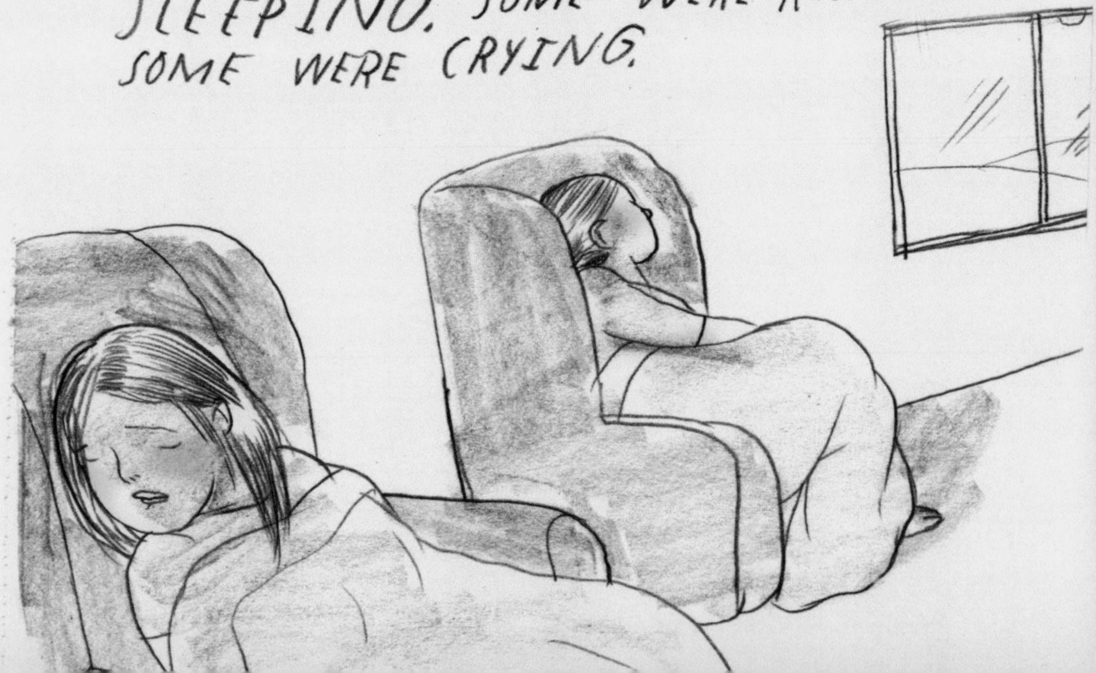

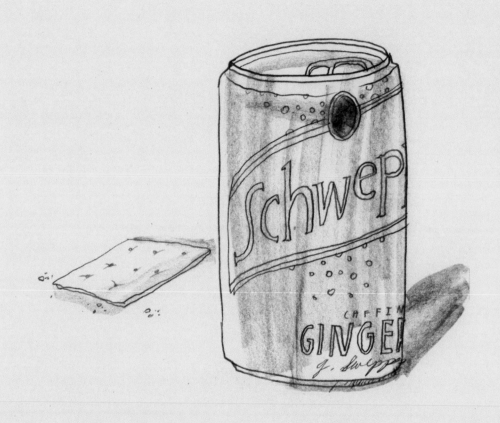

THERE WERE NURSES
WALKING IN AND OFFERING
GINGER ALE AND CRACKERS IN CASE
ANYONE FELT FAINT.

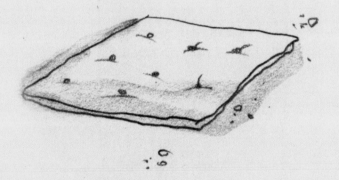

LISA DIDN'T FEEL FAINT OR SICK LIKE SOME OF THE GIRLS DID, BUT SHE DID FEEL CRAMPY AND SORE. SHE ALSO FELT <u>VERY</u> OUT OF IT.

SHE DIDN'T REALLY KNOW HOW LONG SHE RESTED BEFORE SHE WAS GENTLY ESCORTED TO THE DOWNSTAIRS AREA...

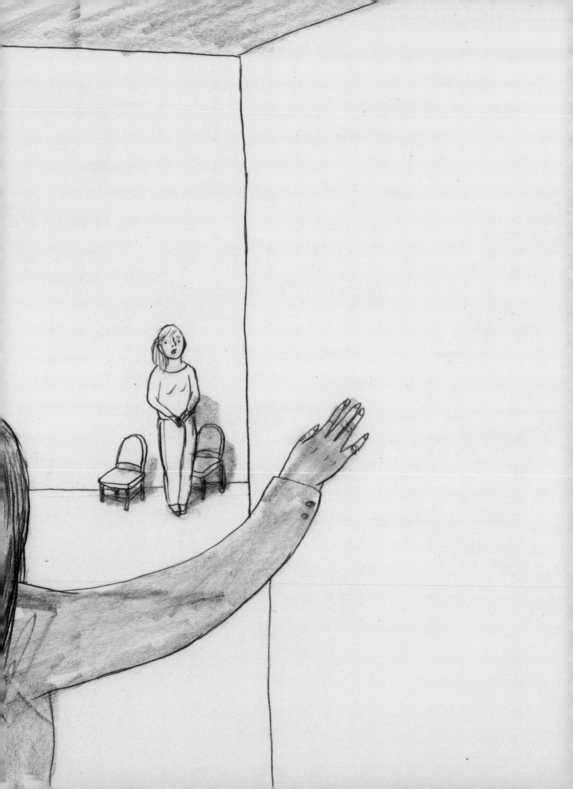

...WHERE HER SISTER WAS
WAITING FOR HER.

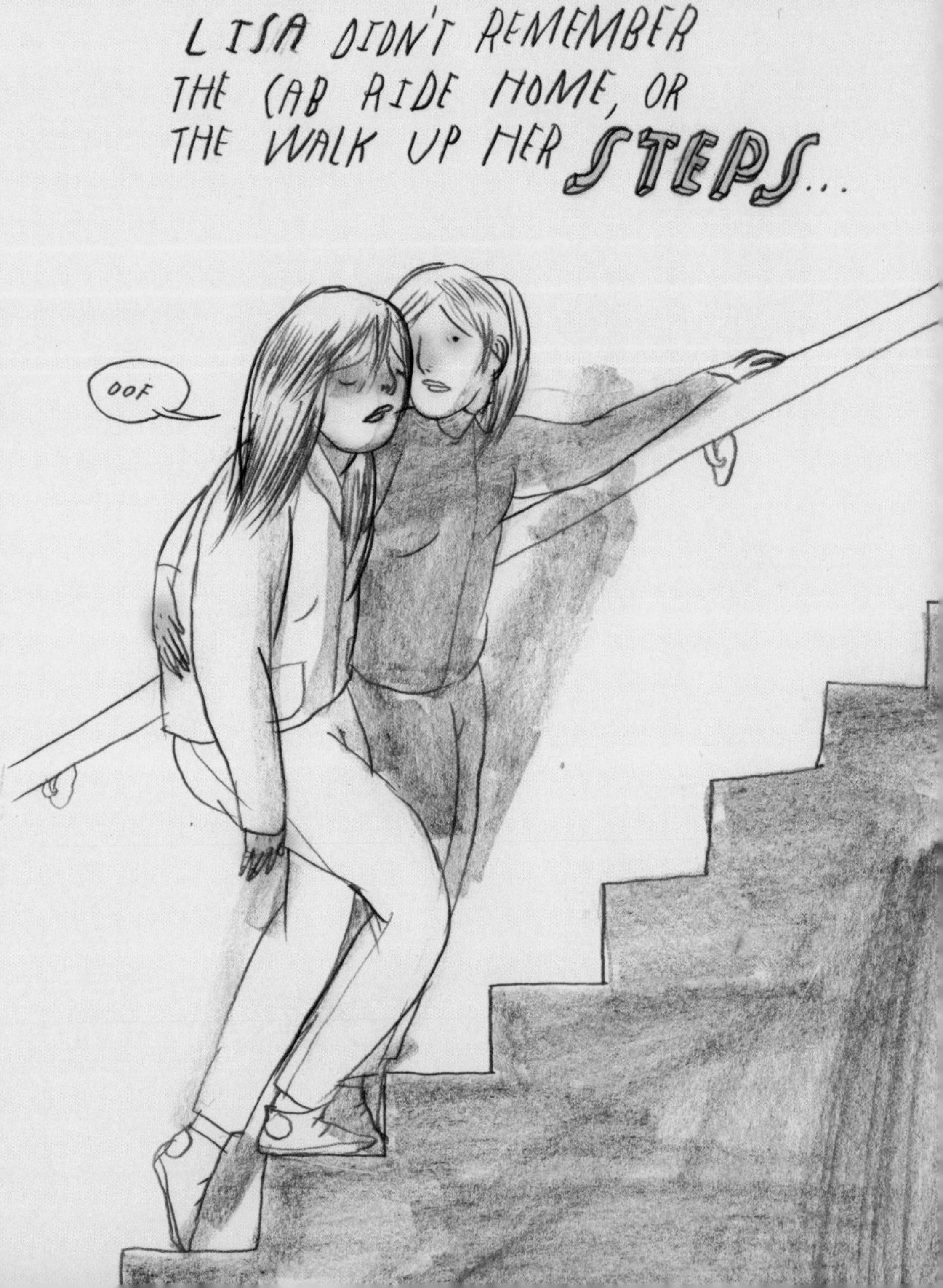
LISA DIDN'T REMEMBER THE CAB RIDE HOME, OR THE WALK UP HER STEPS...
OOF

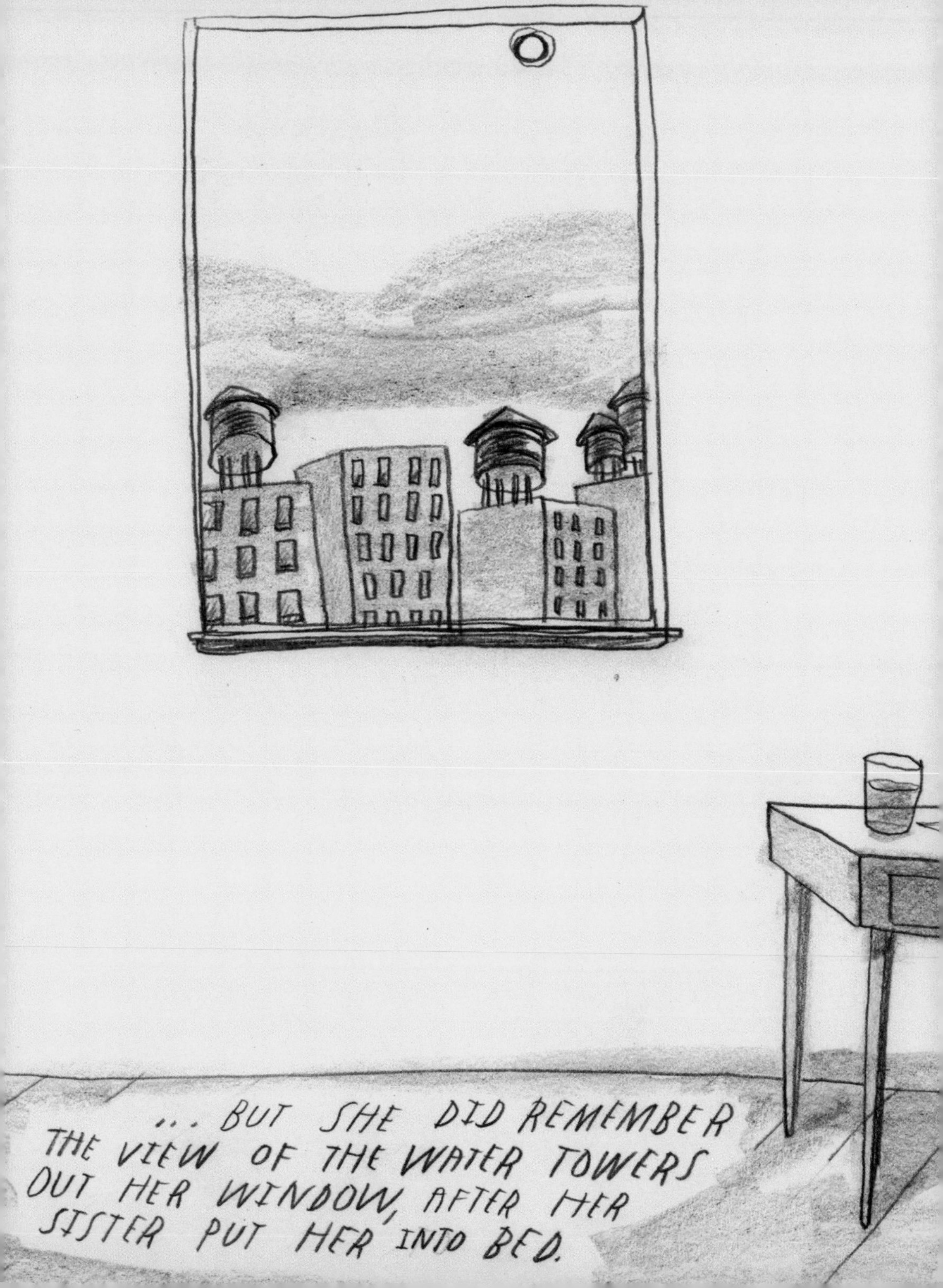
... BUT SHE DID REMEMBER THE VIEW OF THE WATER TOWERS OUT HER WINDOW, AFTER HER SISTER PUT HER INTO BED.

WHEN SHE WOKE
UP THE NEXT MORNING,
LISA FELT VERY SORE,
AND HAD SOME BLEEDING
WHEN SHE WENT TO THE
BATHROOM. KINDA LIKE
A MEDIUM-ISH **PERIOD**.
THE NURSES AT THE CLINIC
HAD GIVEN HER SOME
VERY BIG PADS TO
WEAR OVER THE NEXT FEW
DAYS, IN CASE THE BLEEDING
GOT HEAVIER. SHE FELT LIKE
SHE WAS WEARING A
DIAPER.

THE NURSE HAD ALSO GIVEN
HER INSTRUCTIONS NOT TO
HAVE SEX OR USE TAMPONS
FOR (AT LEAST) SEVERAL WEEKS.

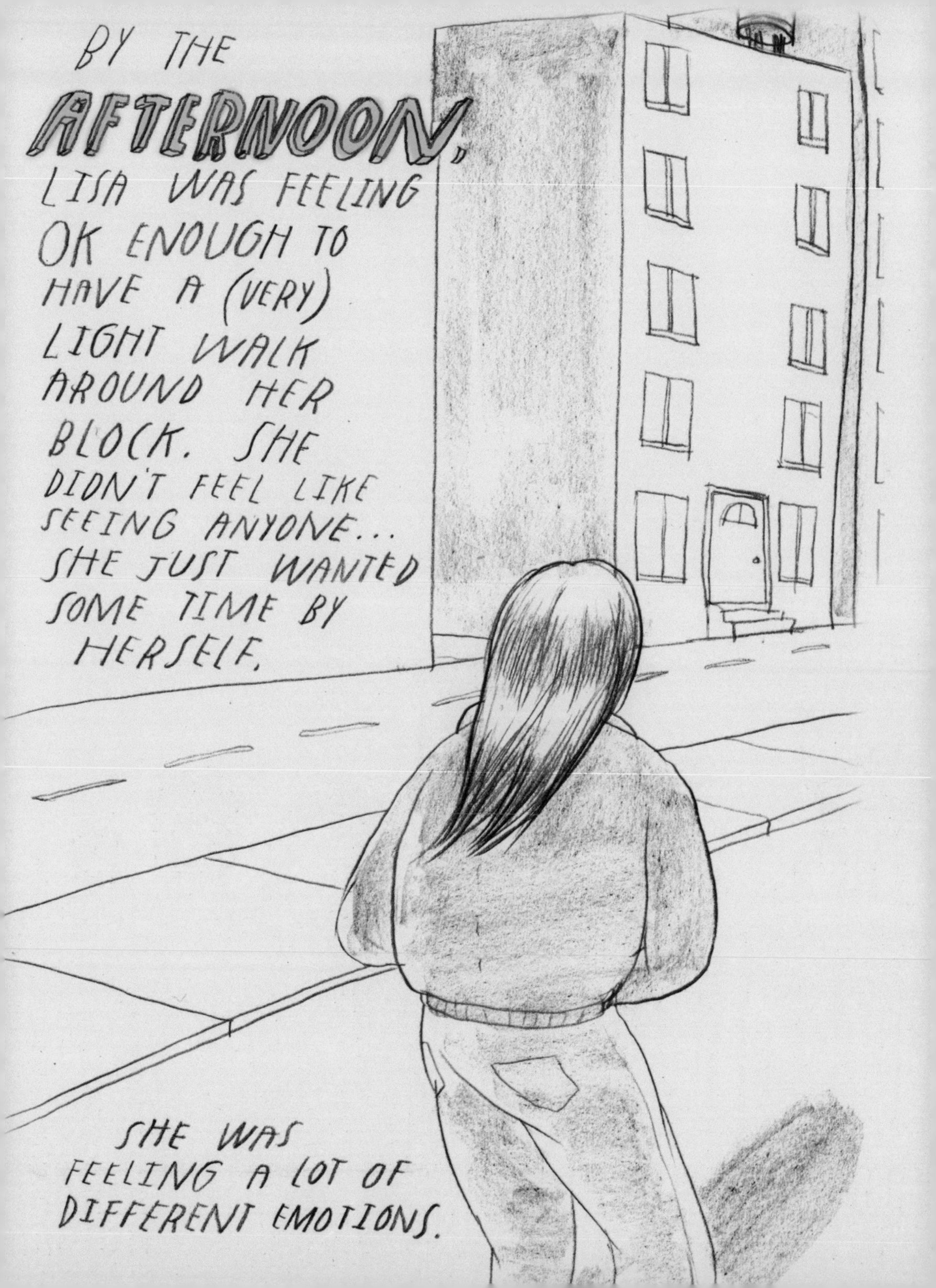
BY THE AFTERNOON, LISA WAS FEELING OK ENOUGH TO HAVE A (VERY) LIGHT WALK AROUND HER BLOCK. SHE DIDN'T FEEL LIKE SEEING ANYONE... SHE JUST WANTED SOME TIME BY HERSELF.
SHE WAS FEELING A LOT OF DIFFERENT EMOTIONS.

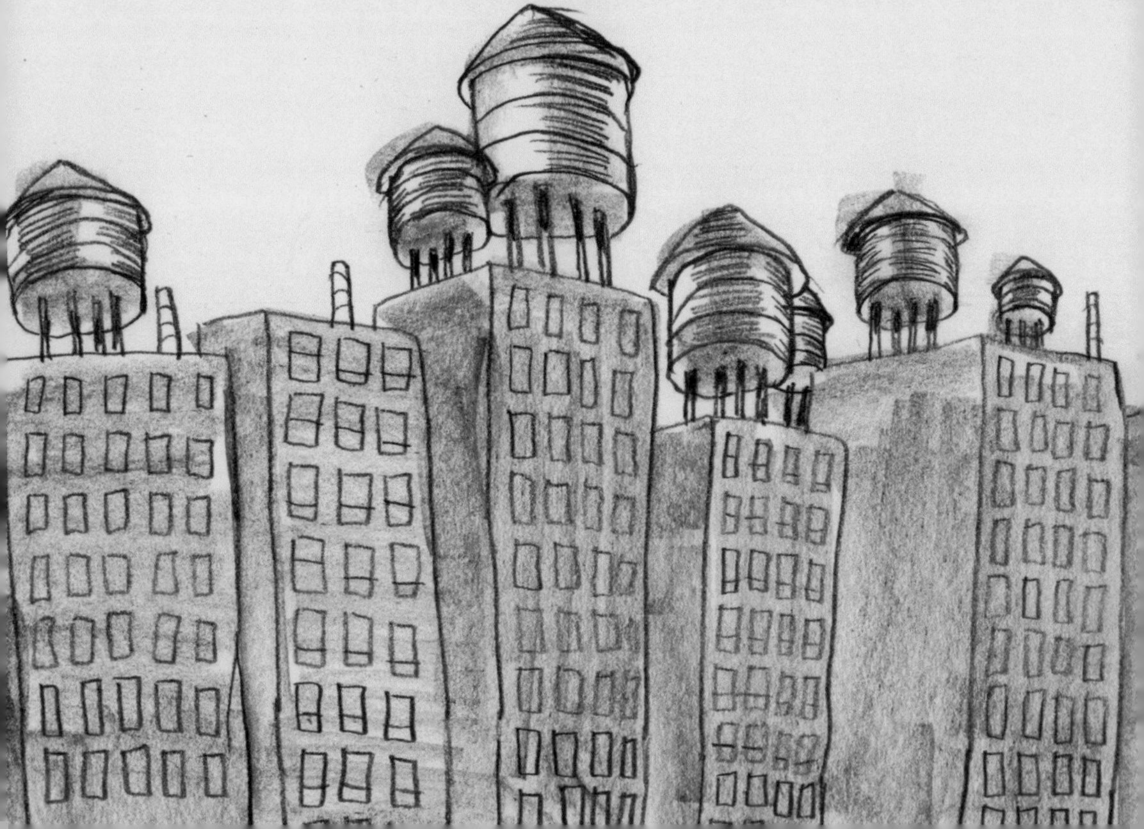

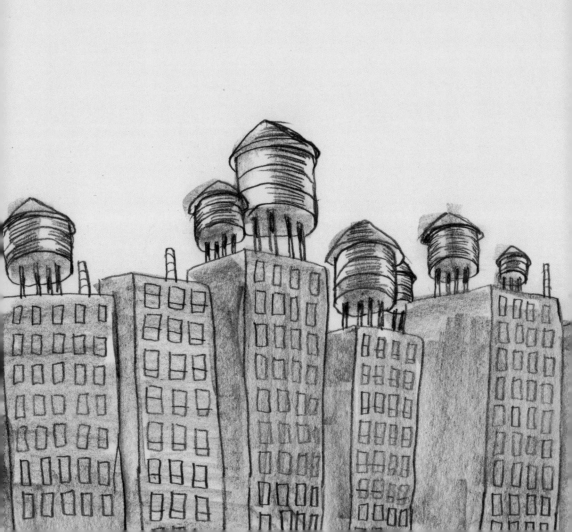

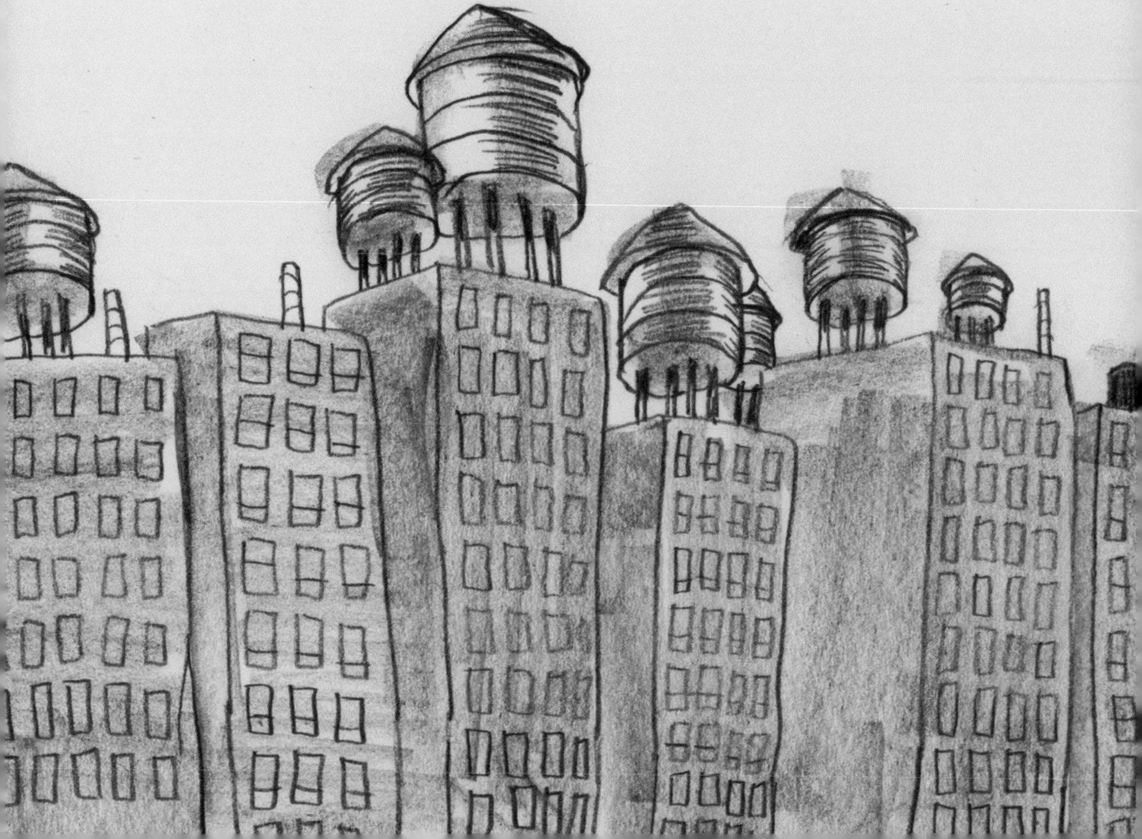

PHYSICAL RECOVERY
FROM AN ABORTION
CAN BE VERY FAST.

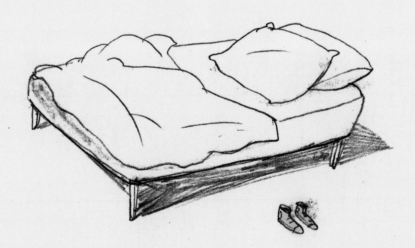

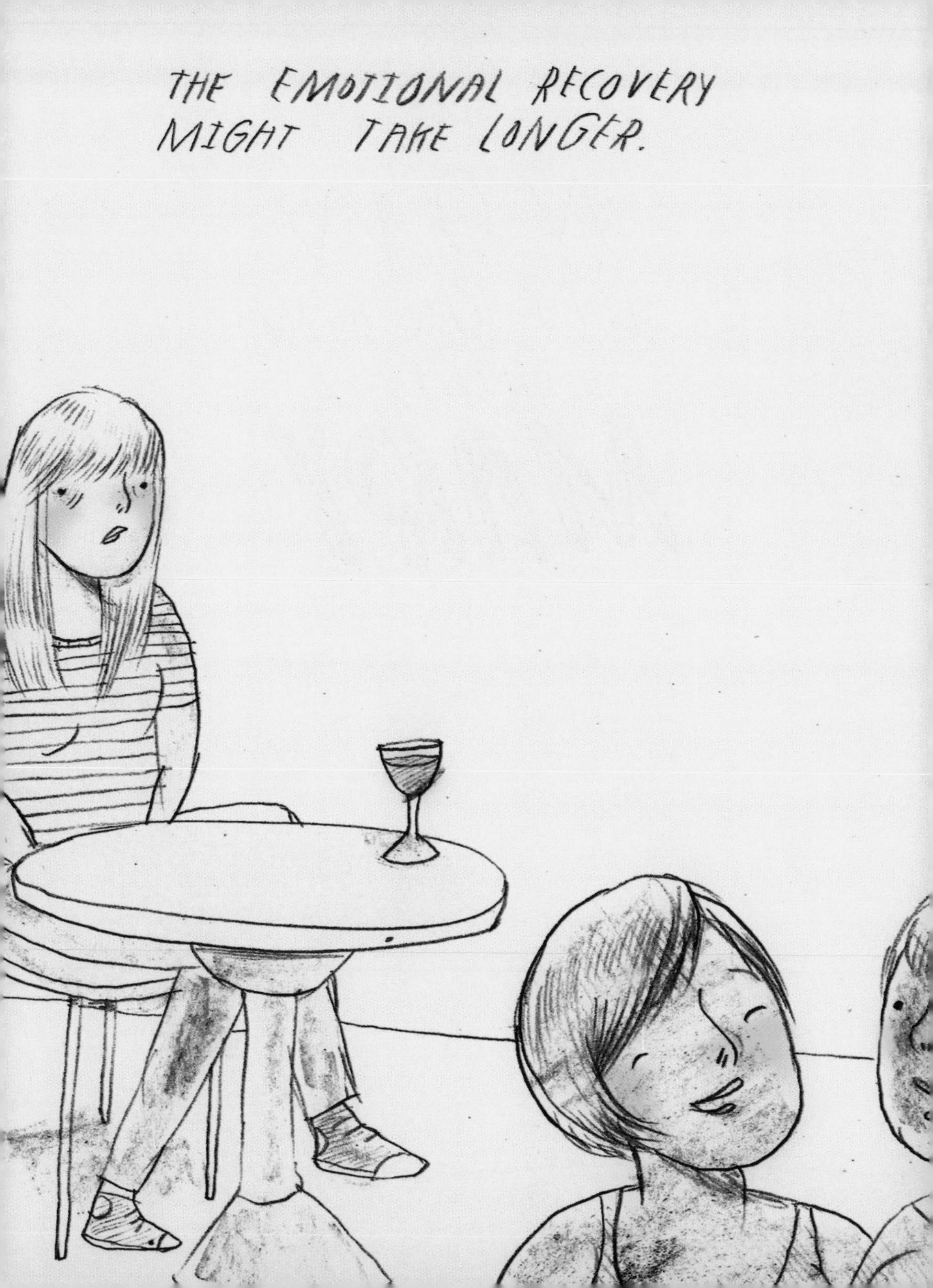
THE EMOTIONAL RECOVERY MIGHT TAKE LONGER.

N O W

LET'S CHECK IN

WITH

MARY.

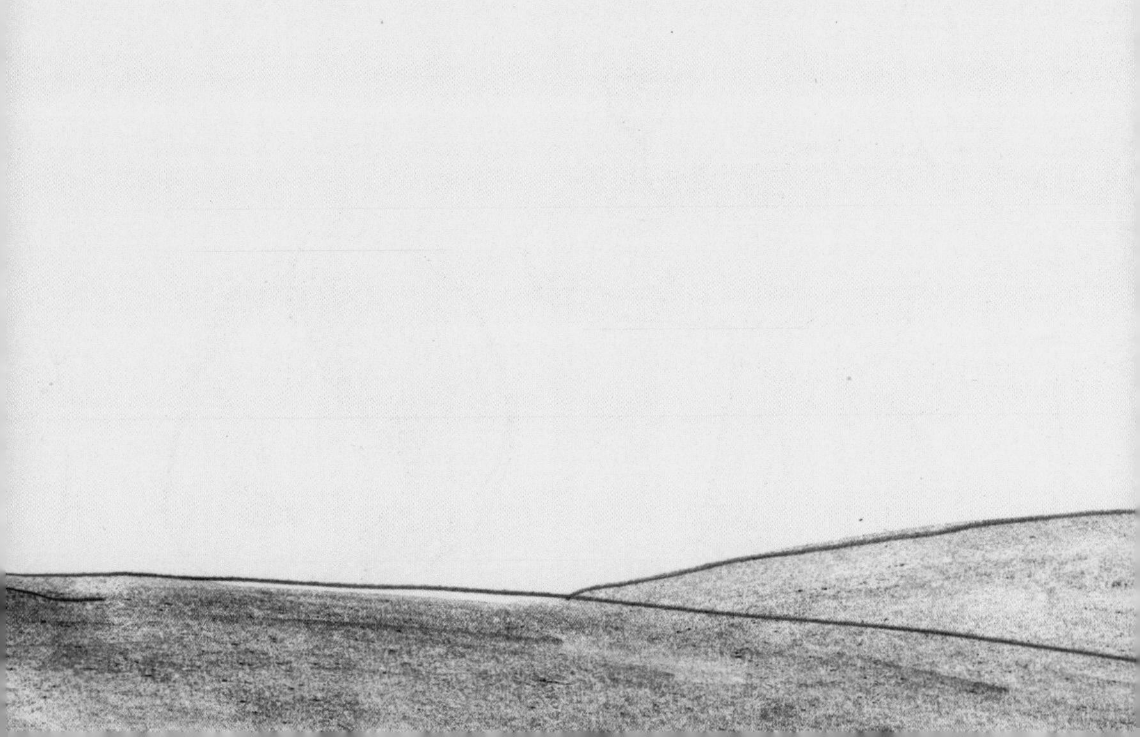

MARY WASN'T A FAN OF HOSPITALS. SO WHEN SHE CALLED THE CLINIC AND THEY TOLD HER THAT (BASED ON HOW FAR ALONG IN HER PREGNANCY SHE THOUGHT SHE WAS) SHE HAD THE OPTION OF TAKING THE PILL-FORM

AT HOME...

SHE DECIDED TO GO WITH THAT.

HOSPITALS JUST SMELL WEIRD TO ME, I GUESS.

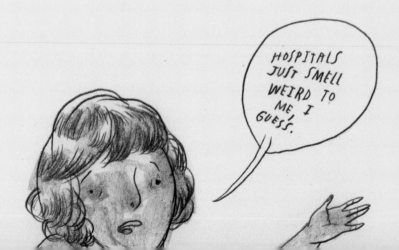

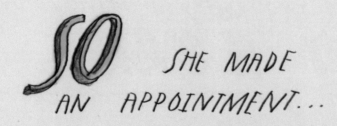

SO SHE MADE AN APPOINTMENT...

...AND LIKE LISA, WAS A LITTLE NERVOUS. SHE WASN'T SURE WHAT TO EXPECT.

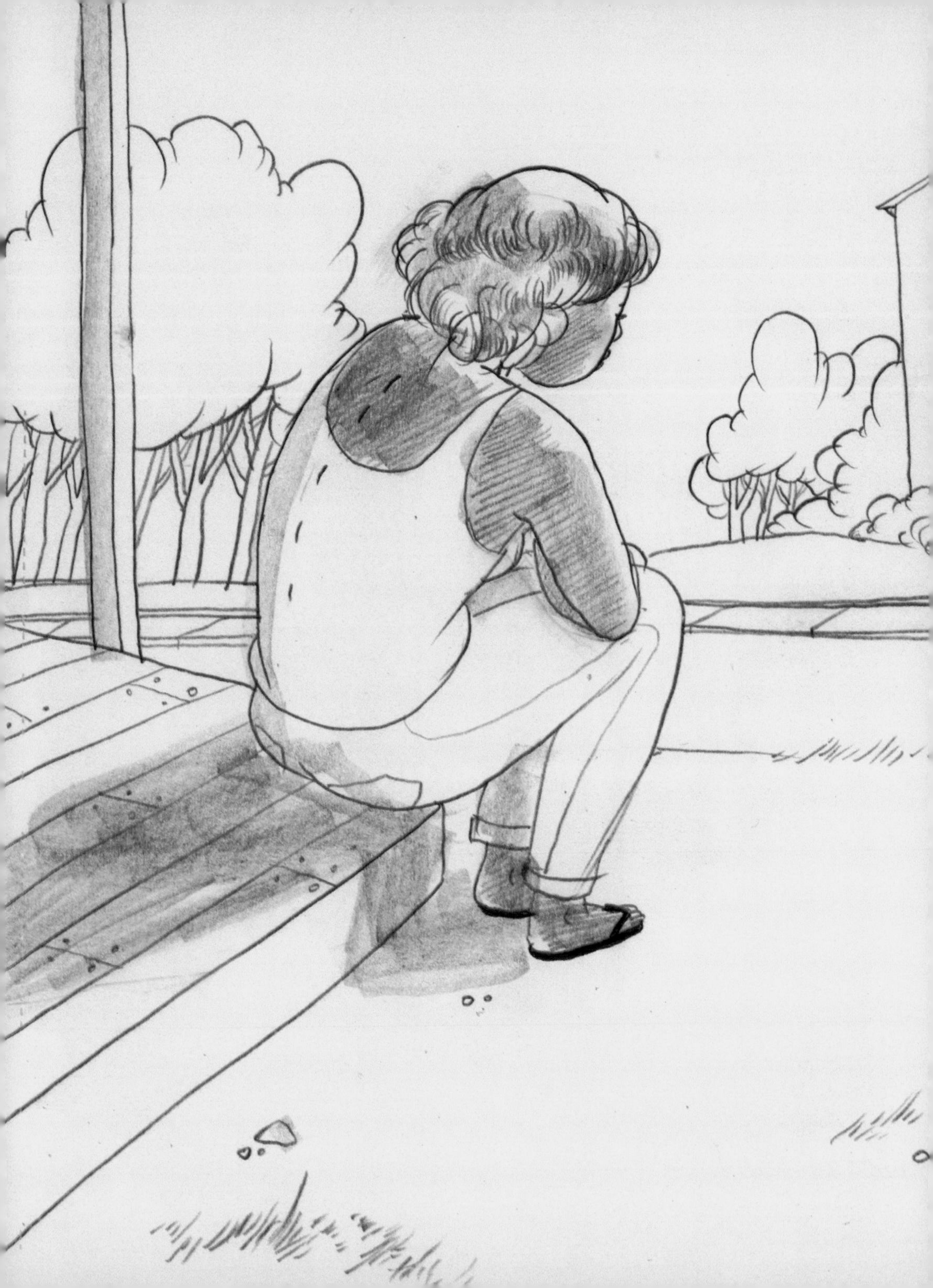

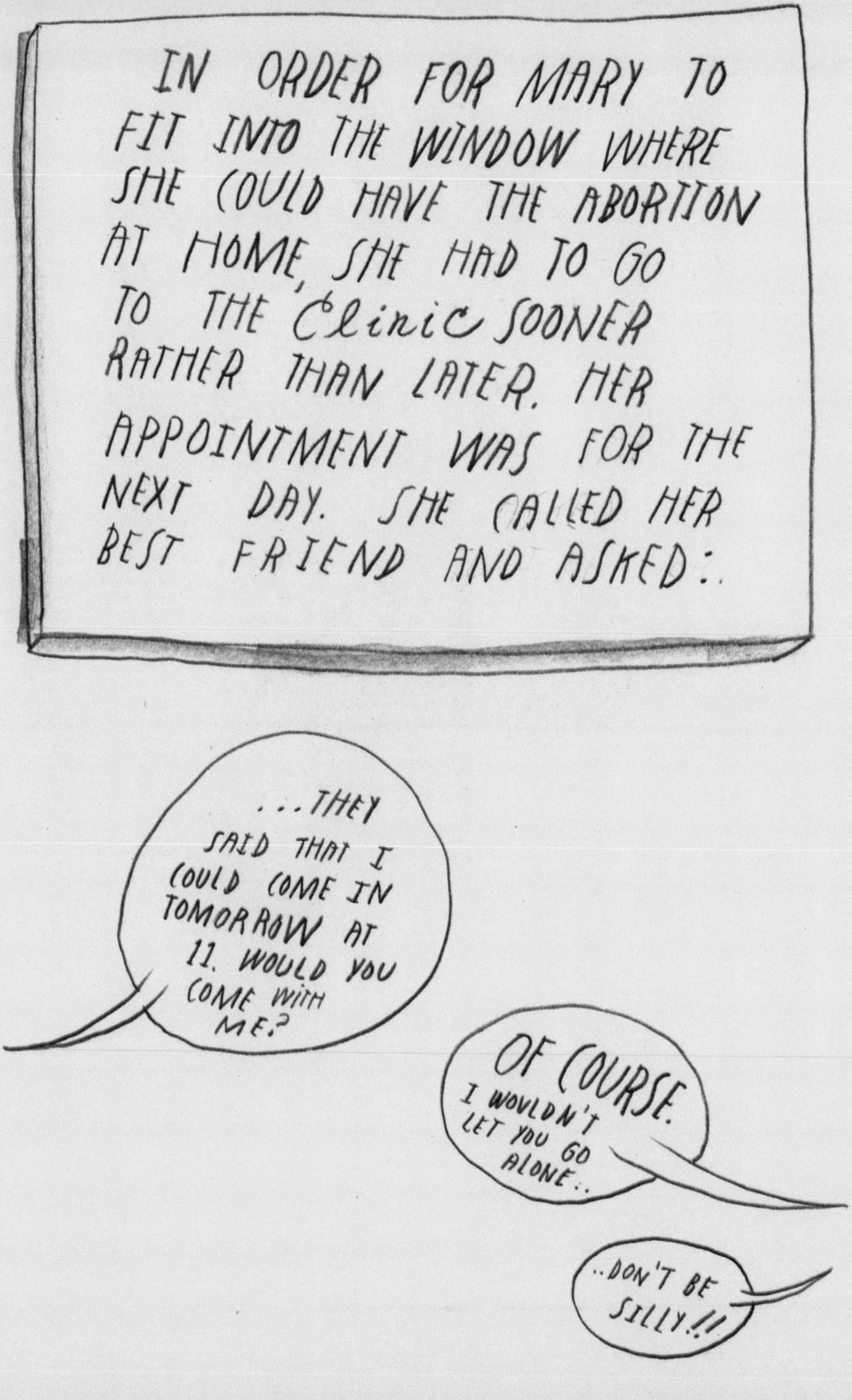
IN ORDER FOR MARY TO FIT INTO THE WINDOW WHERE SHE COULD HAVE THE ABORTION AT HOME, SHE HAD TO GO TO THE Clinic SOONER RATHER THAN LATER. HER APPOINTMENT WAS FOR THE NEXT DAY. SHE CALLED HER BEST FRIEND AND ASKED:..
...THEY SAID THAT I COULD COME IN TOMORROW AT 11. WOULD YOU COME WITH ME?
OF COURSE. I WOULDN'T LET YOU GO ALONE..
..DON'T BE SILLY!!!

IN THE MORNING, MARY WAS READY. HER FRIEND PICKED HER UP AND THEY DROVE TO THE CLINIC. THEY CHATTED AND LAUGHED, BUT MARY WAS NERVOUS.

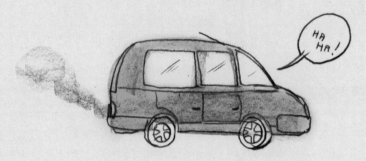

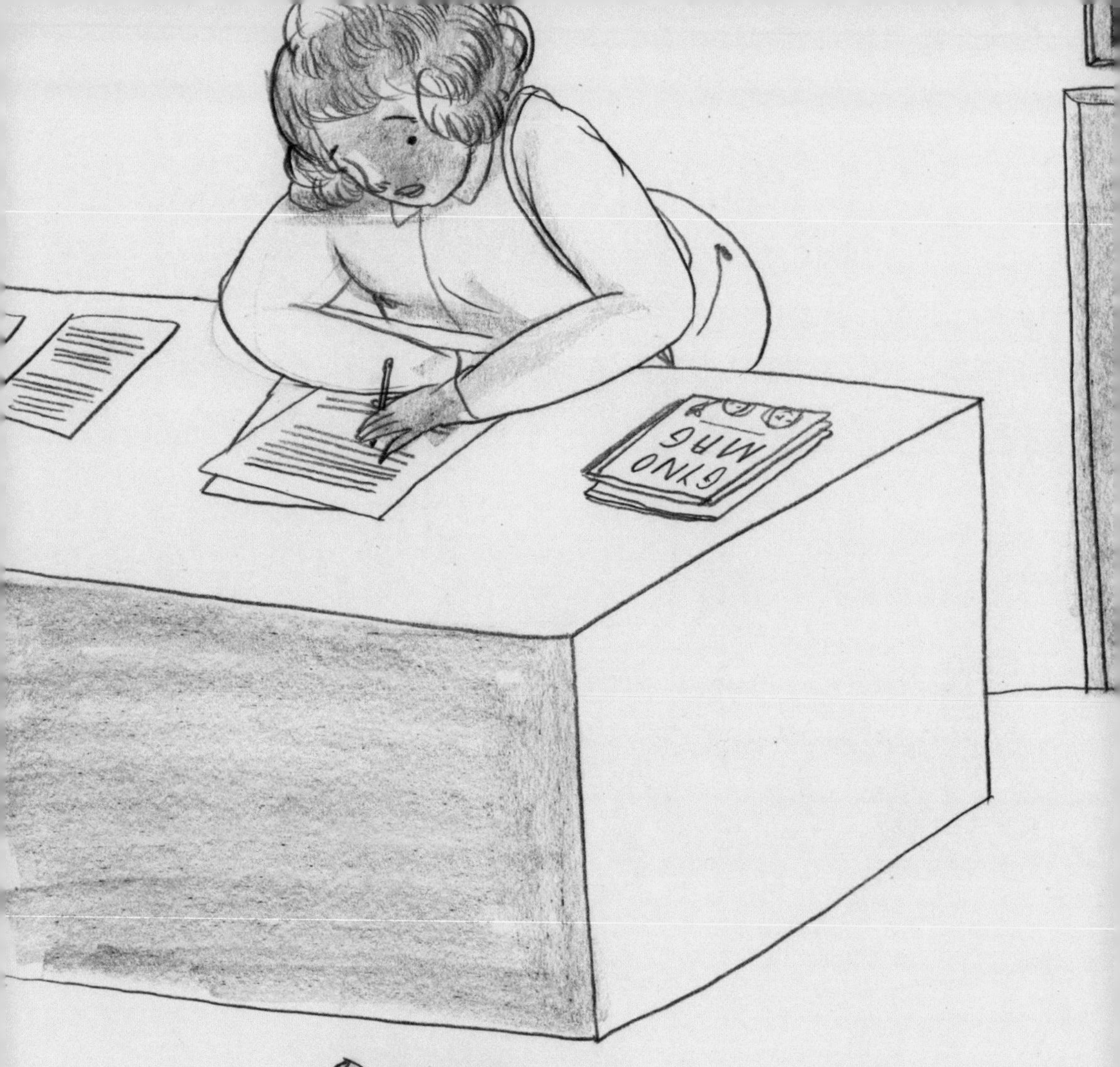
GYNO MAG

JUST LIKE LISA, MARY HAD TO FILL OUT A LOT OF PAPERWORK, PAY UP FRONT, AND WAIT IN THE WAITING ROOM BEFORE SEEING A DOCTOR. EVENTUALLY THEY CALLED HER NAME.

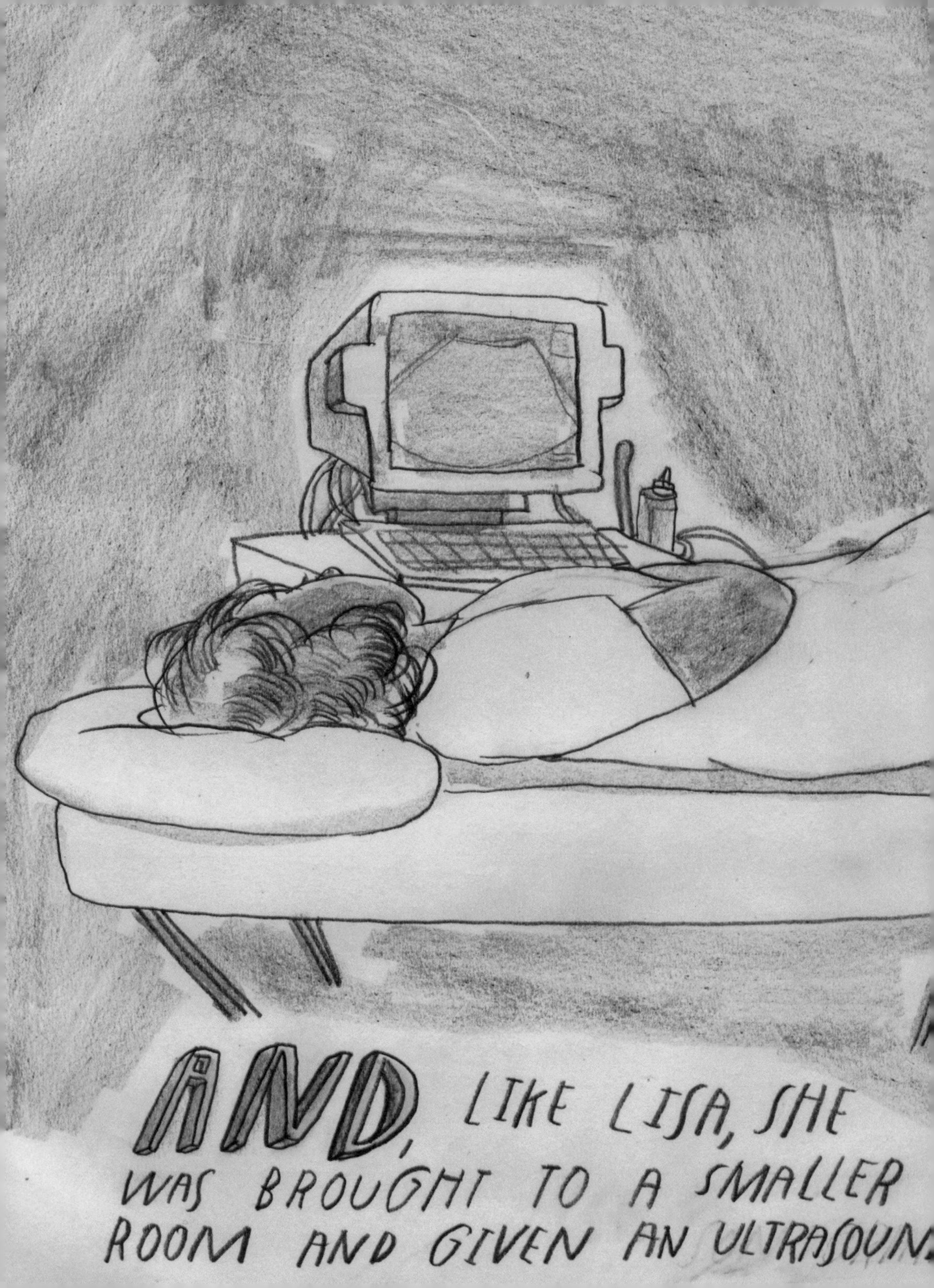
AND, LIKE LISA, SHE
WAS BROUGHT TO A SMALLER
ROOM AND GIVEN AN ULTRASOUN

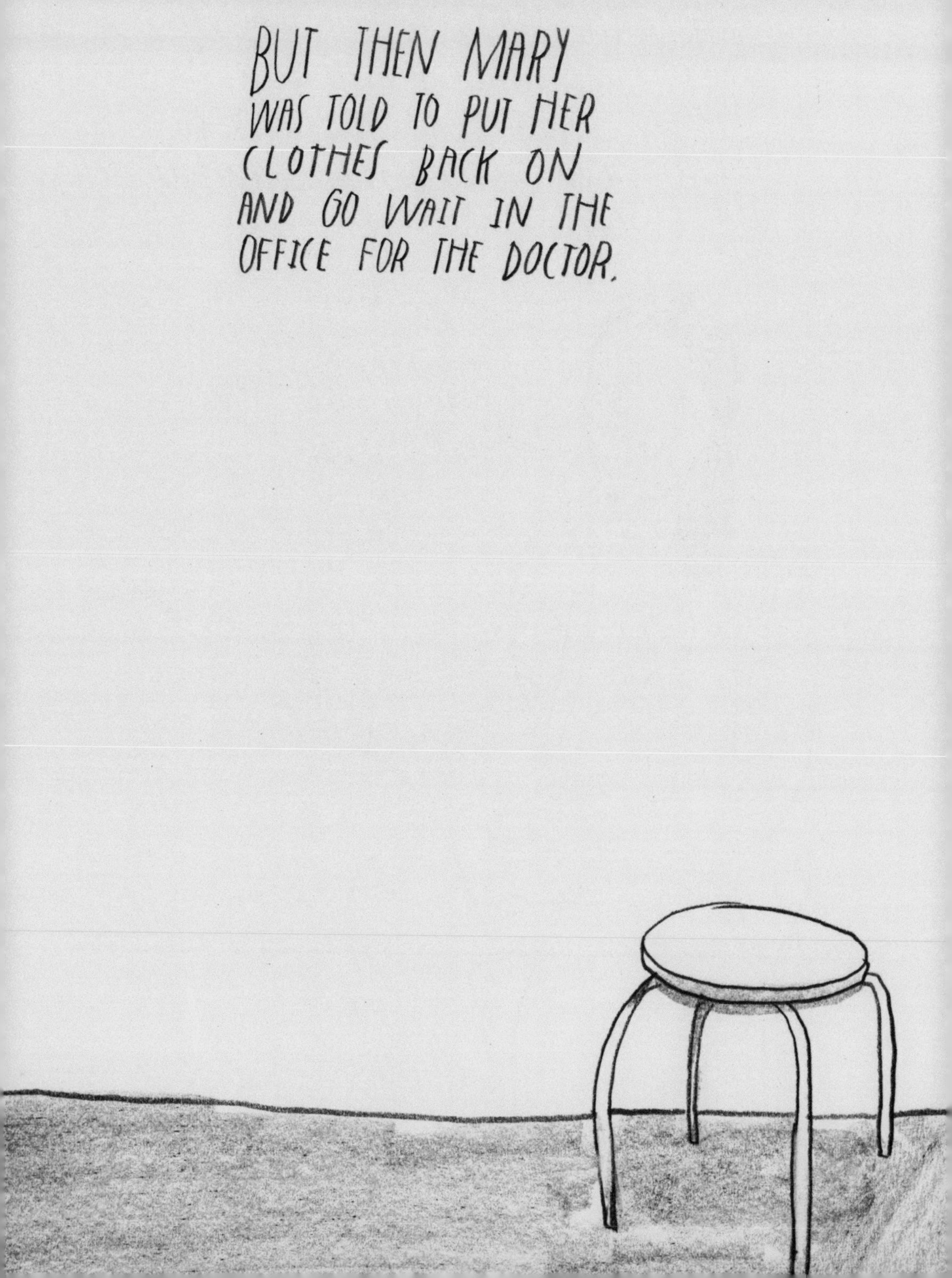
BUT THEN MARY WAS TOLD TO PUT HER CLOTHES BACK ON AND GO WAIT IN THE OFFICE FOR THE DOCTOR.

WHEN THE DOCTOR CAME IN, SHE EXPLAINED WHAT WAS GOING TO HAPPEN TO MARY OVER THE NEXT HOURS (AND DAYS) AFTER LEAVING THE CLINIC.

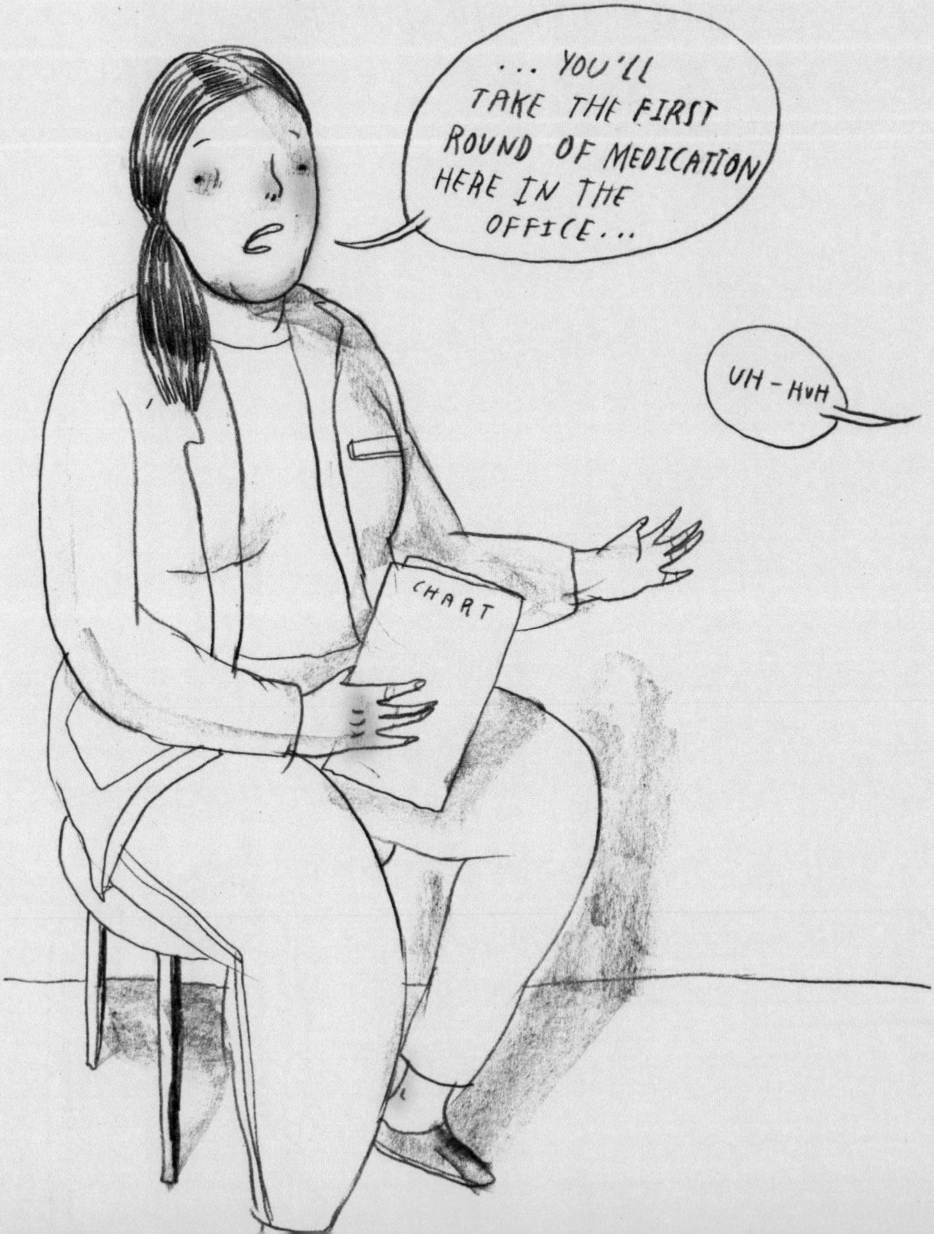
... YOU'LL TAKE THE FIRST ROUND OF MEDICATION HERE IN THE OFFICE...
UH-HUH
CHART

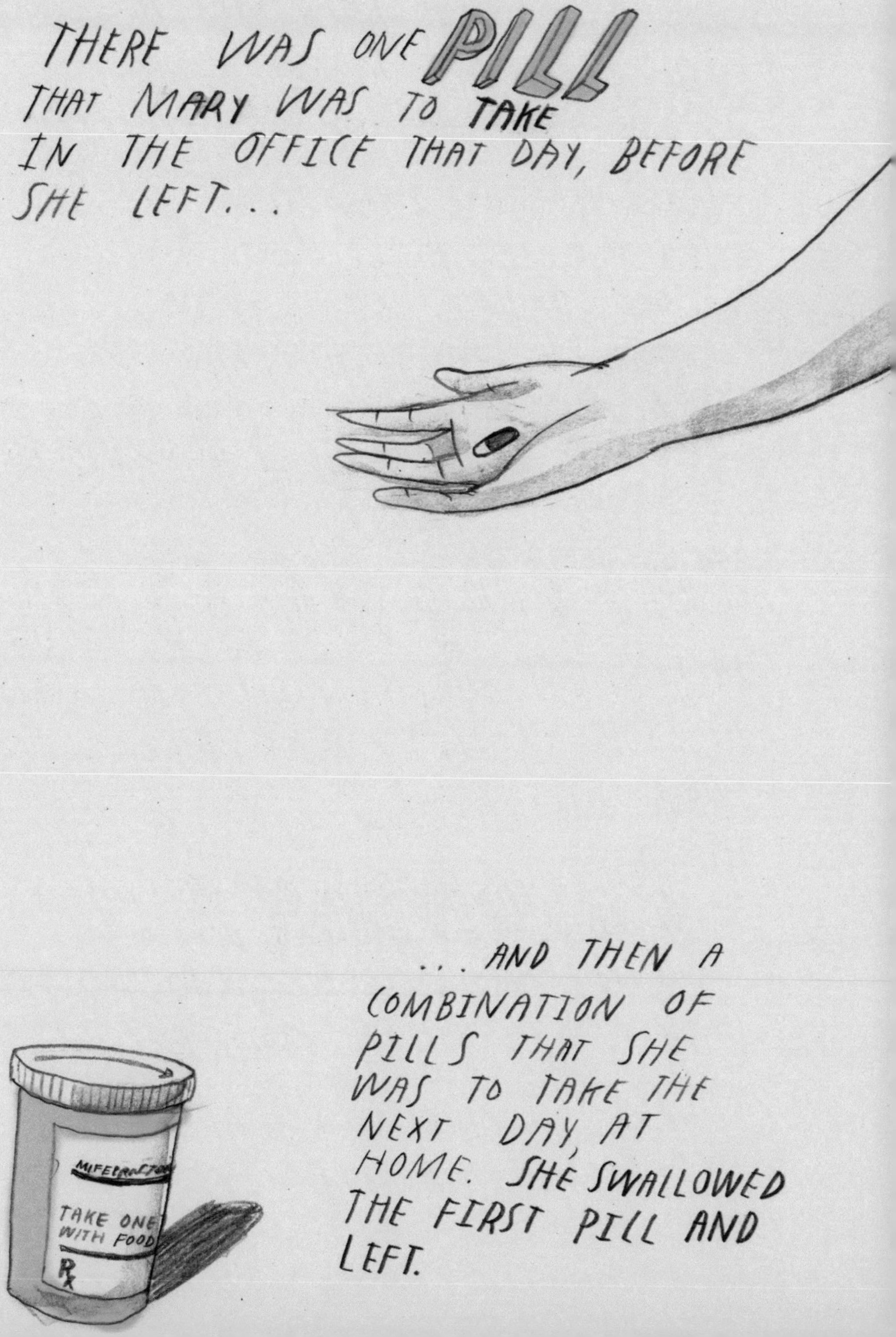
THERE WAS ONE PILL THAT MARY WAS TO TAKE IN THE OFFICE THAT DAY, BEFORE SHE LEFT...
...AND THEN A COMBINATION OF PILLS THAT SHE WAS TO TAKE THE NEXT DAY, AT HOME. SHE SWALLOWED THE FIRST PILL AND LEFT.
TAKE ONE WITH FOOD
Rx

IN CASE YOU'D LIKE A REMINDER... A "MEDICAL" ABORTION IS THE PROCESS OF ENDING THE PREGNANCY WITH THE USE OF PILLS. ONE OF THE MOST COMMON MEDICATIONS USED IS A COMBINATION OF

MIFEPRISTONE

(AND)

MISOPROSTOL.

MIFEPRISTONE (THE FIRST PILL TAKEN AT THE OFFICE) BLOCKS PROGESTERONE FROM THE UTERINE LINING, STOPPING THE **PREGNANCY** FROM CONTINUING, WHILE MISOPROSTOL (TAKEN 24 TO 48 HOURS LATER) CAUSES CONTRACTIONS THAT EXPEL THE FETUS.

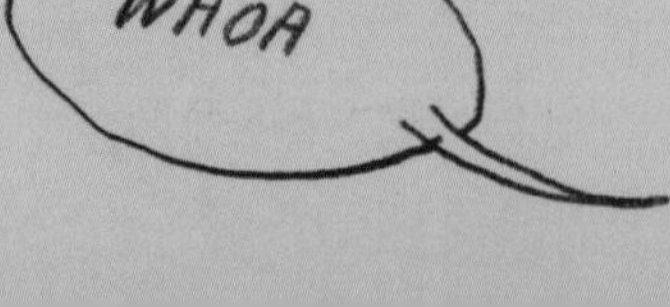
WHOA

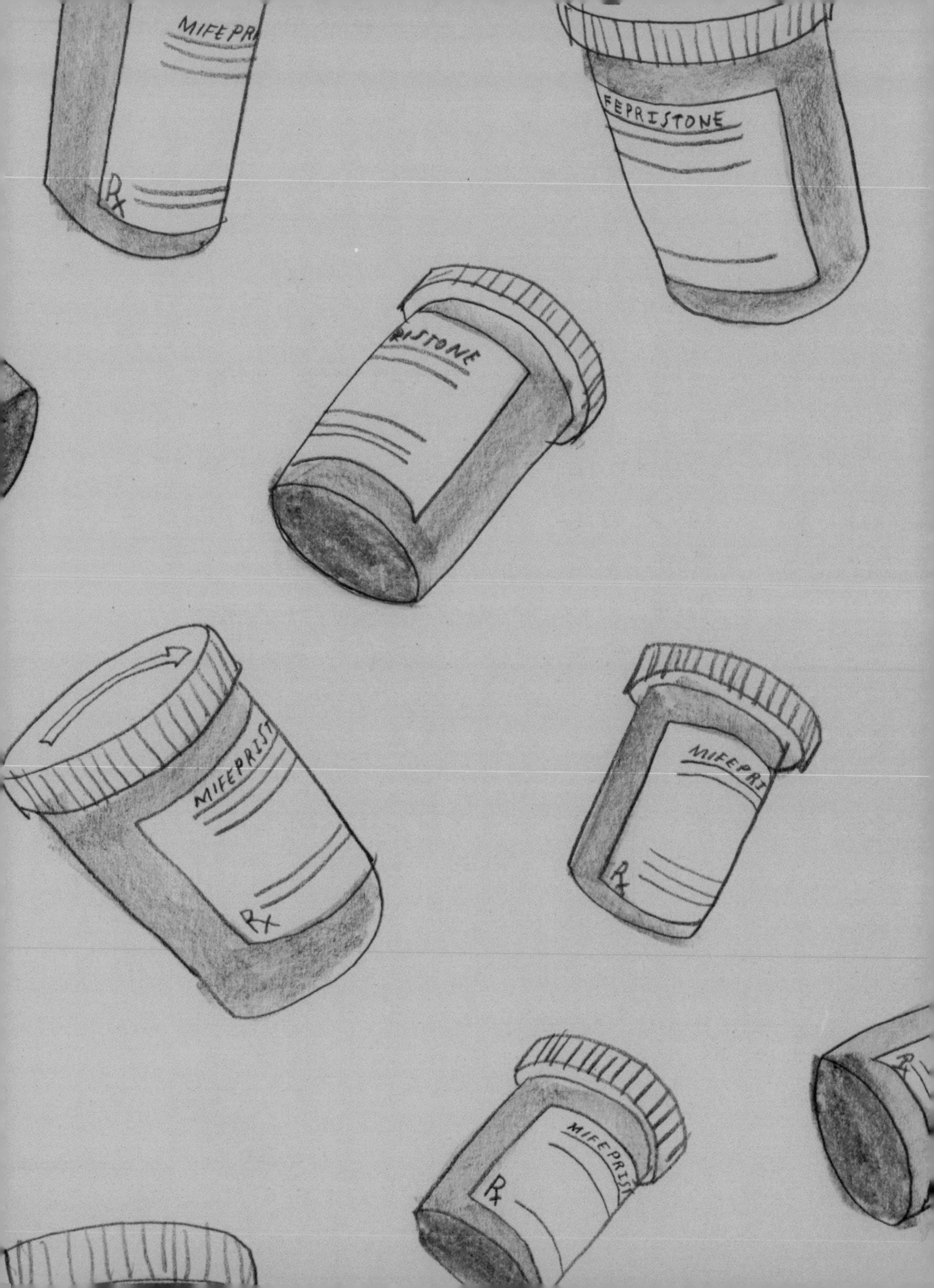
MIFEPRI
Rx
FEPRISTONE
RISTONE
MIFEPRIST
Rx
MIFEPRI
Rx
MIFEPRIST
Rx

MARY'S FRIEND DROVE
HER HOME AND THEY SAT ON
THE COUCH AND TALKED. SHE
DID NOT FEEL ANYTHING
STRANGE . . . THE DOCTOR HAD
TOLD HER THE SHE MAY OR MAY
NOT FEEL ANYTHING UNTIL SHE
TOOK THE SECOND MEDICATION, THE
MISOPROSTOL. AFTER A WHILE SHE
DECIDED TO TAKE A WALK.

CAN WE WATCH STAR WARS?

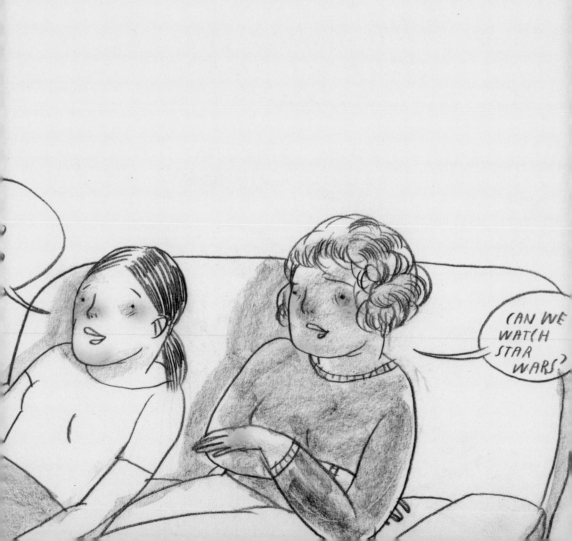

SHE WONDERED WHEN IT
WOULD ALL START TO
HAPPEN.

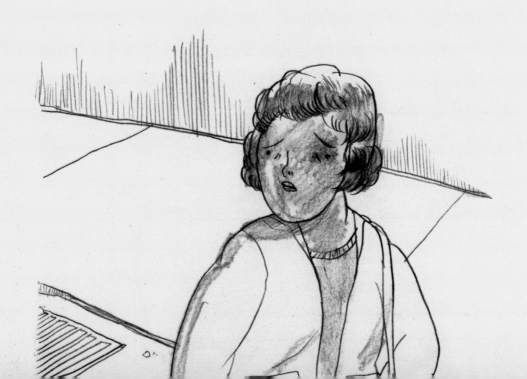

AS IT TURNED OUT, MARY HARDLY FELT ANYTHING FROM THE FIRST PILL. AT THE TIME INDICATED, SHE EVENTUALLY TOOK THE MISOPROSTOL. SHE CALLED HER FRIEND (WHO HAD GONE HOME TO FEED HER CAT), AND ASKED HER TO COME BACK.

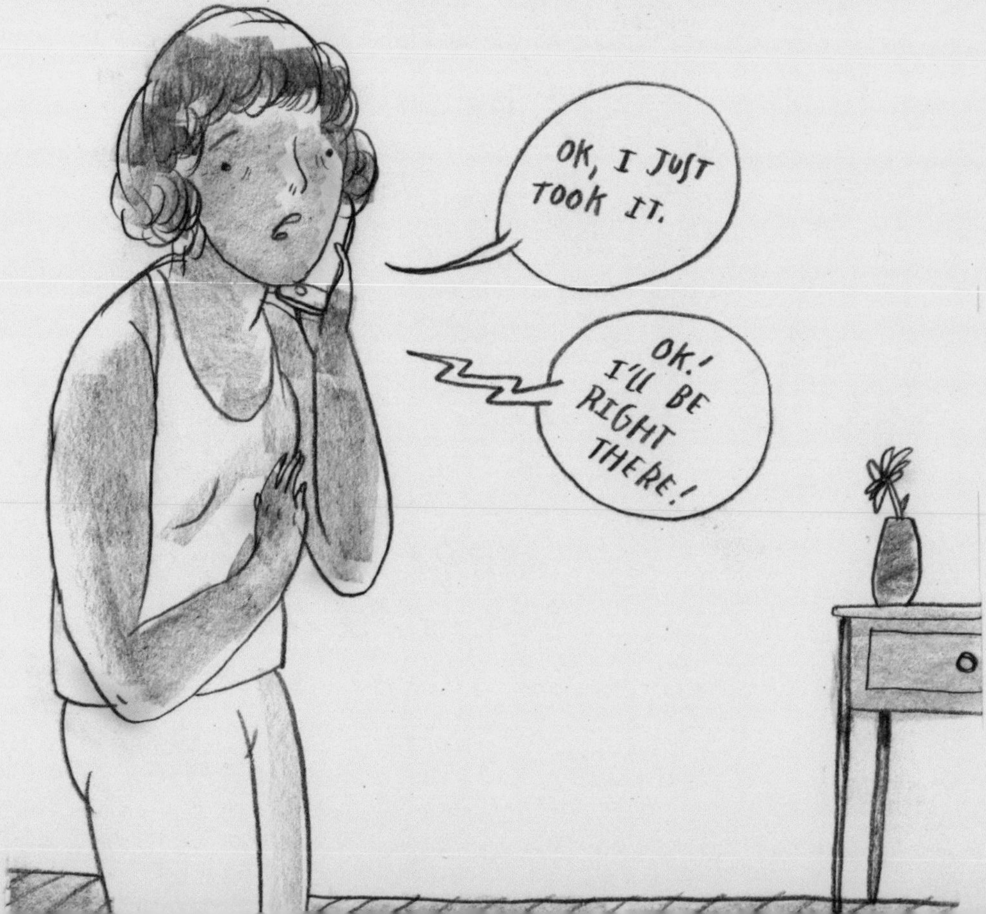
OK, I JUST TOOK IT.
OK! I'LL BE RIGHT THERE!

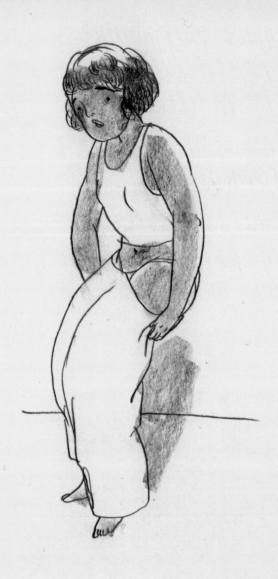

MARY GOT INTO
HER PAJAMAS...

... AND SET HERSELF UP
ON THE COUCH WITH
SOME MAGAZINES.

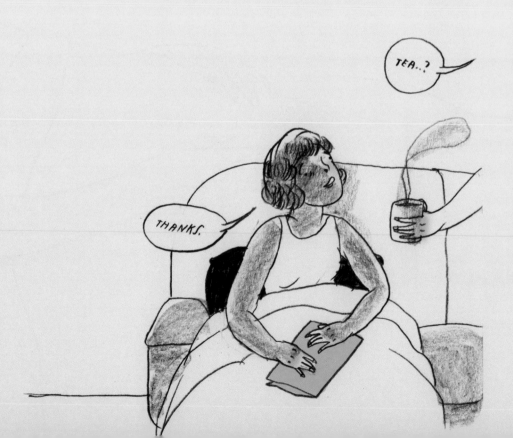

AFTER

ABOUT AN HOUR,
SHE BEGAN TO FEEL
CRAMPS, LIKE A
PERIOD. THEY
WERE PRETTY STRONG.

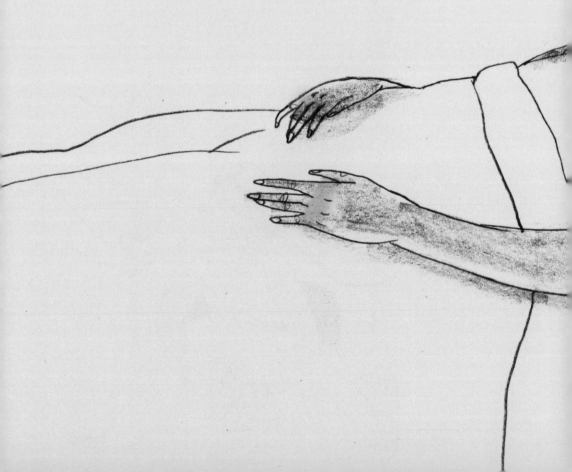

THEN SHE FELT NAUSEOUS, AND SHE THREW UP. IN A LOT OF WAYS, THIS WAS THE WORST PART. MARY HATED THROWING UP.

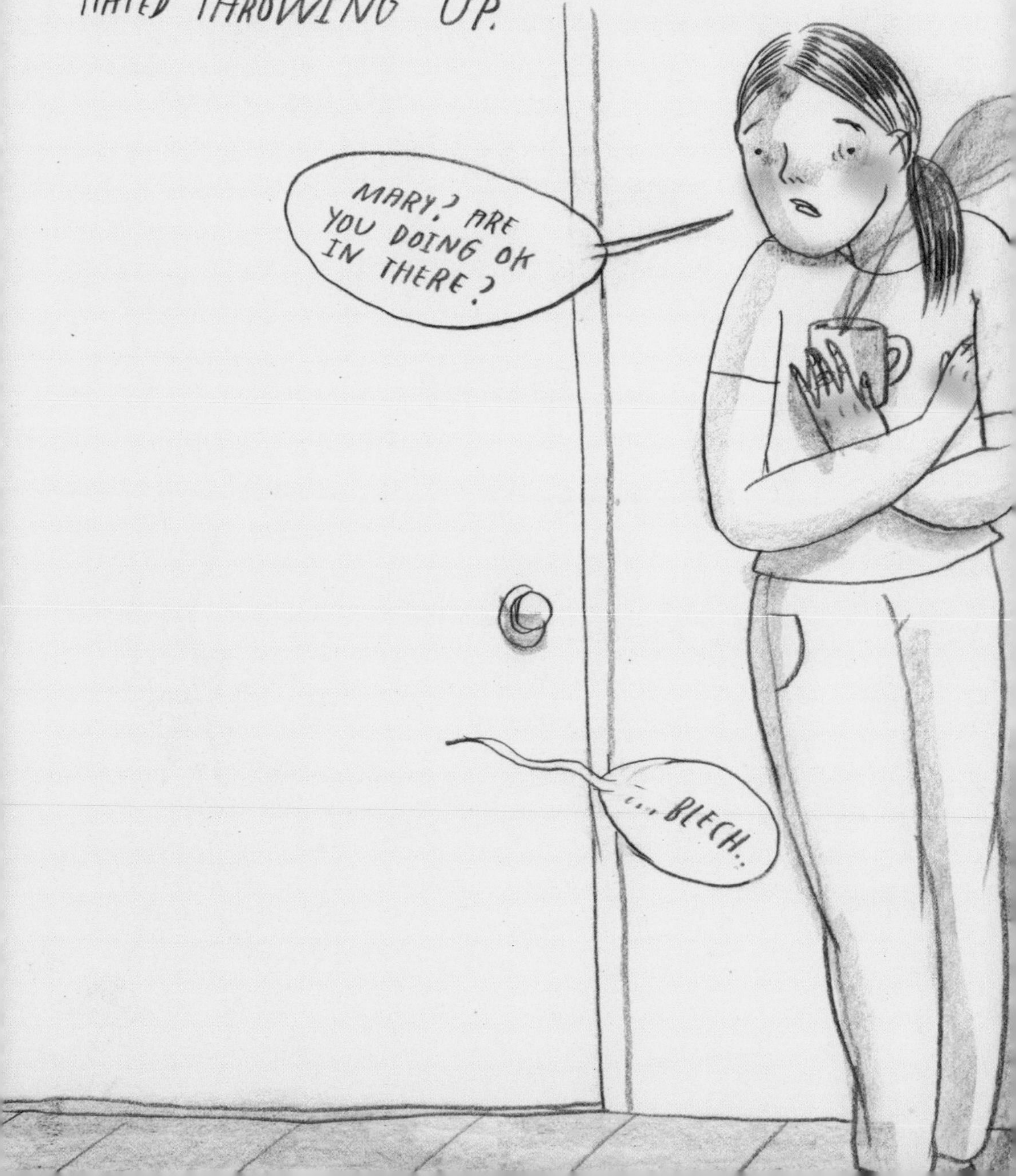
MARY? ARE YOU DOING OK IN THERE?
...BLECH..

EVERYTHING SHE WAS FEELING WAS WHAT THE DOCTOR HAD TOLD HER TO EXPECT. THEY HAD EVEN GIVEN HER A SHEET OF PAPER WITH IT ALL WRITTEN OUT:

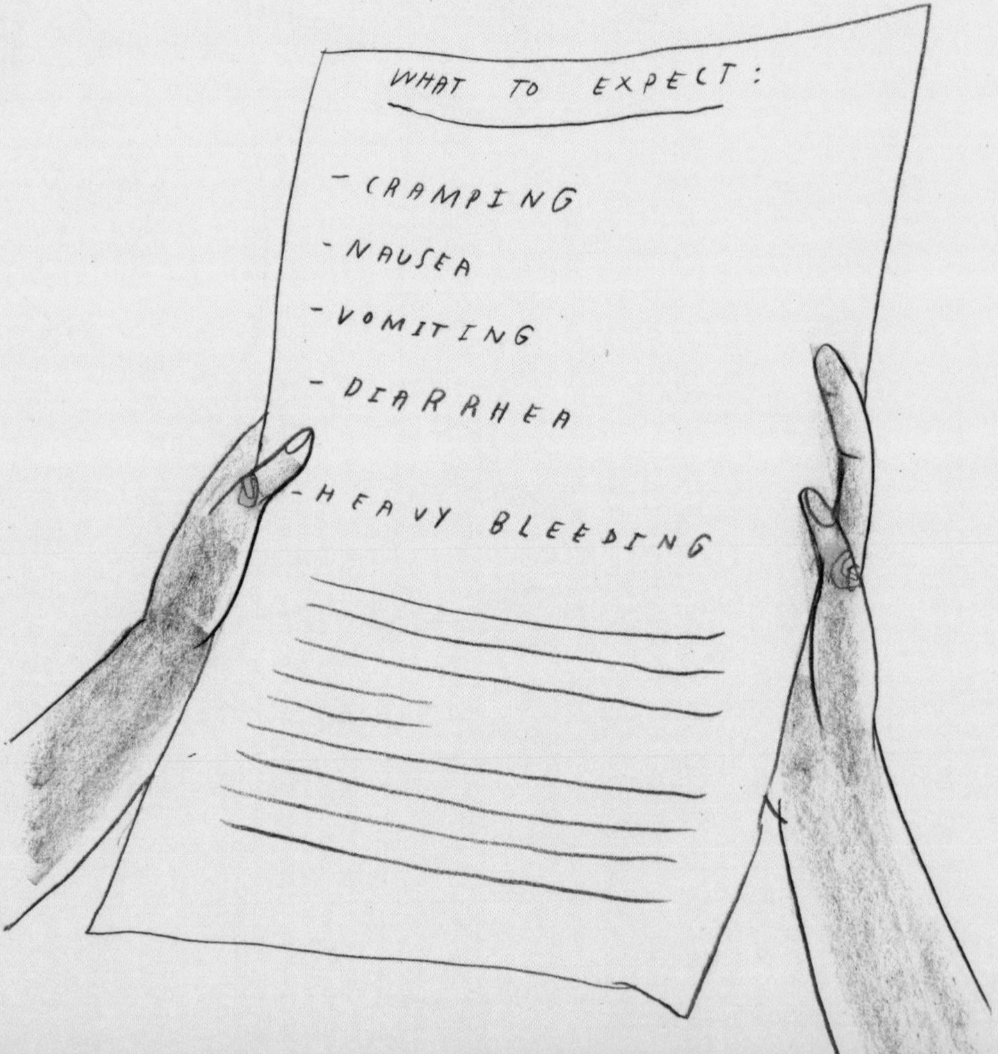
WHAT TO EXPECT:
-CRAMPING
-NAUSEA
-VOMITING
-DIARRHEA
-HEAVY BLEEDING

SIDE NOTE!
SIDE NOTE!
SIDE NOTE!
SIDE NOTE!
SIDE NOTE!

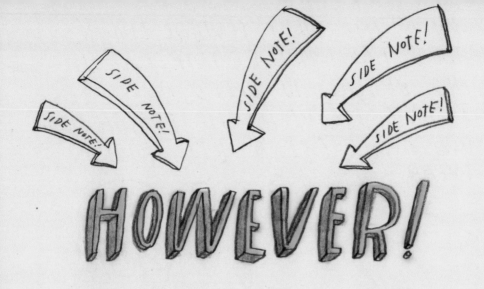

HOWEVER!

THE DOCTOR, A PIECE OF PAPER, THE INTERNET, YOUR FRIENDS, OR THIS BOOK CANNOT TELL YOU HOW LONG THE PROCESS WILL TAKE. IT WILL TAKE HOW-EVER LONG IT WILL TAKE (AND YOU WILL FEEL BETTER AFTER IT'S DONE, DON'T WORRY).* MOST WOMEN ABORT WITHIN 4 OR FIVE HOURS AFTER TAKING MISOPROSTOL. SOMETIMES IT TAKES LONGER.

*AND SOMETIMES (A VERY SMALL PERCENT OF THE TIME), THE PROCEDURE IS NOT SUCCESSFUL AT EXPELLING THE FETUS, AND YOU MUST THEN HAVE A SURGICAL ABORTION.

OVER THE NEXT SEVERAL HOURS, MARY HAD MORE CRAMPING. SHE HAD BEGUN TO BLEED, AND IT BECAME HEAVIER. THE DOCTOR HAD GIVEN HER EXTRA-BIG PADS TO WEAR.

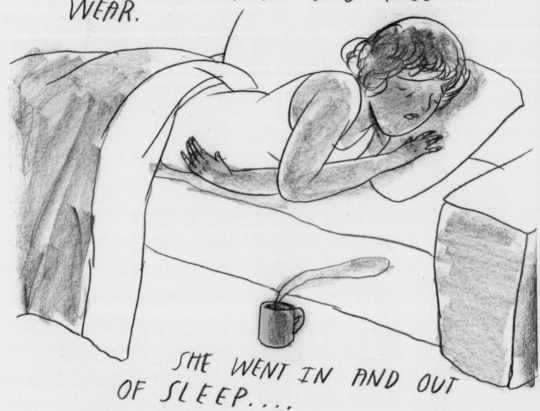

SHE WENT IN AND OUT OF SLEEP....

...IN AND OUT OF DREAMS...

...AND IN AND OUT OF THE BATHROOM TO CHANGE PADS. THERE WAS A LOT OF BLOOD.

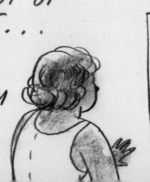

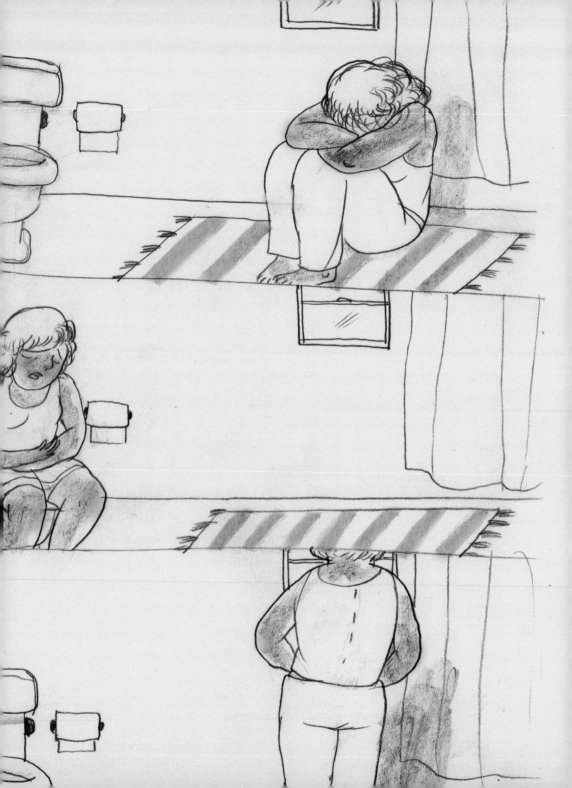

AT ONE POINT, THE BLEEDING GOT VERY HEAVY ALL AT ONCE. SHE KNEW THAT THIS MEANT THAT THE ABORTION HAD REALLY HAPPENED. IT WAS INTENSE AND MADE HER A LITTLE SAD. SHE DIDN'T KNOW WHY.

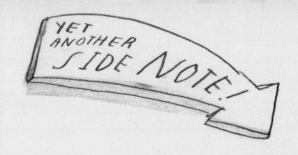

YET ANOTHER SIDE NOTE!

IT IS NORMAL TO HAVE A LOT OF BLEEDING, AND IT IS ALSO NORMAL TO SEE LARGER BLOOD CLOTS. THIS MAY SEEM SCARY, BUT IT'S ACTUALLY A SIGN THAT THE ABORTION IS TAKING PLACE. AFTER A FEW HOURS, THE BLEEDING SHOULD LESSEN.

DON'T BE SCARED IF YOU FEEL:

CRAMPS

DIZZINESS

CHILLS

HEADACHE

NAUSEA

FEVER *

* BUT PLEASE CALL A PHYSICIAN RIGHT AWAY IF ANY OF THESE SYMPTOMS SEEM TO BE LASTING LONGER THAN NORMAL.

MARY FELT SOME OR
ALL OF THESE THINGS OVER
THE COURSE OF THE
AFTERNOON. DURING THE DAY
HER FRIEND BROUGHT HER
WATER AND TEA, READ HER
THE NEWSPAPER, AND HELD
HER HAND WHEN THE CRAMPS
CAME ON STRONG. WHEN
MARY DOZED OFF, HER FRIEND
SAT BESIDE HER AND READ A
BOOK.

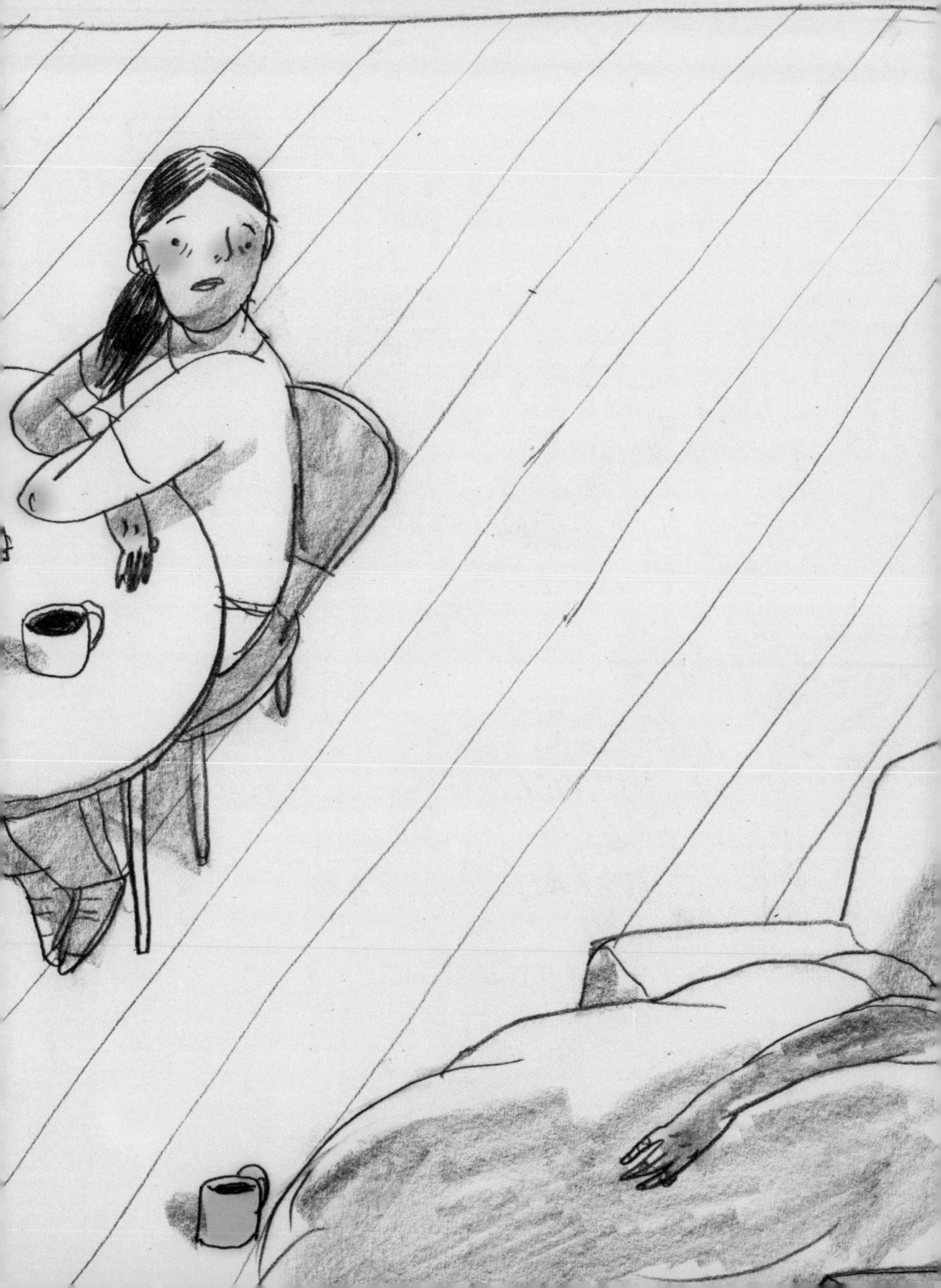

MARY DRIFTED
IN AND OUT
OF SLEEP.
SHE LOST TRACK
OF TIME, ALTHO
ONCE SHE
OPENED HER EYES
AND SAW THAT
THE DAY HAD
TURNED TO NIGHT.
THE BLEEDING
WAS SLOWING
DOWN, TOO.

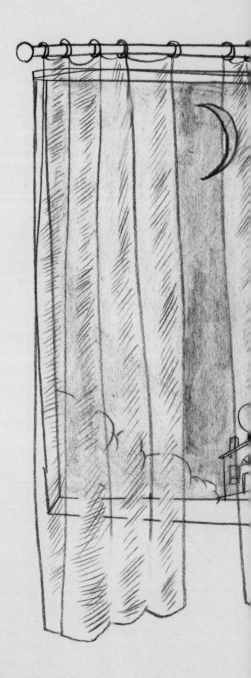

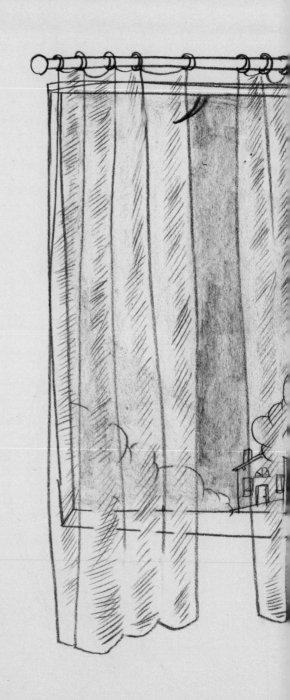

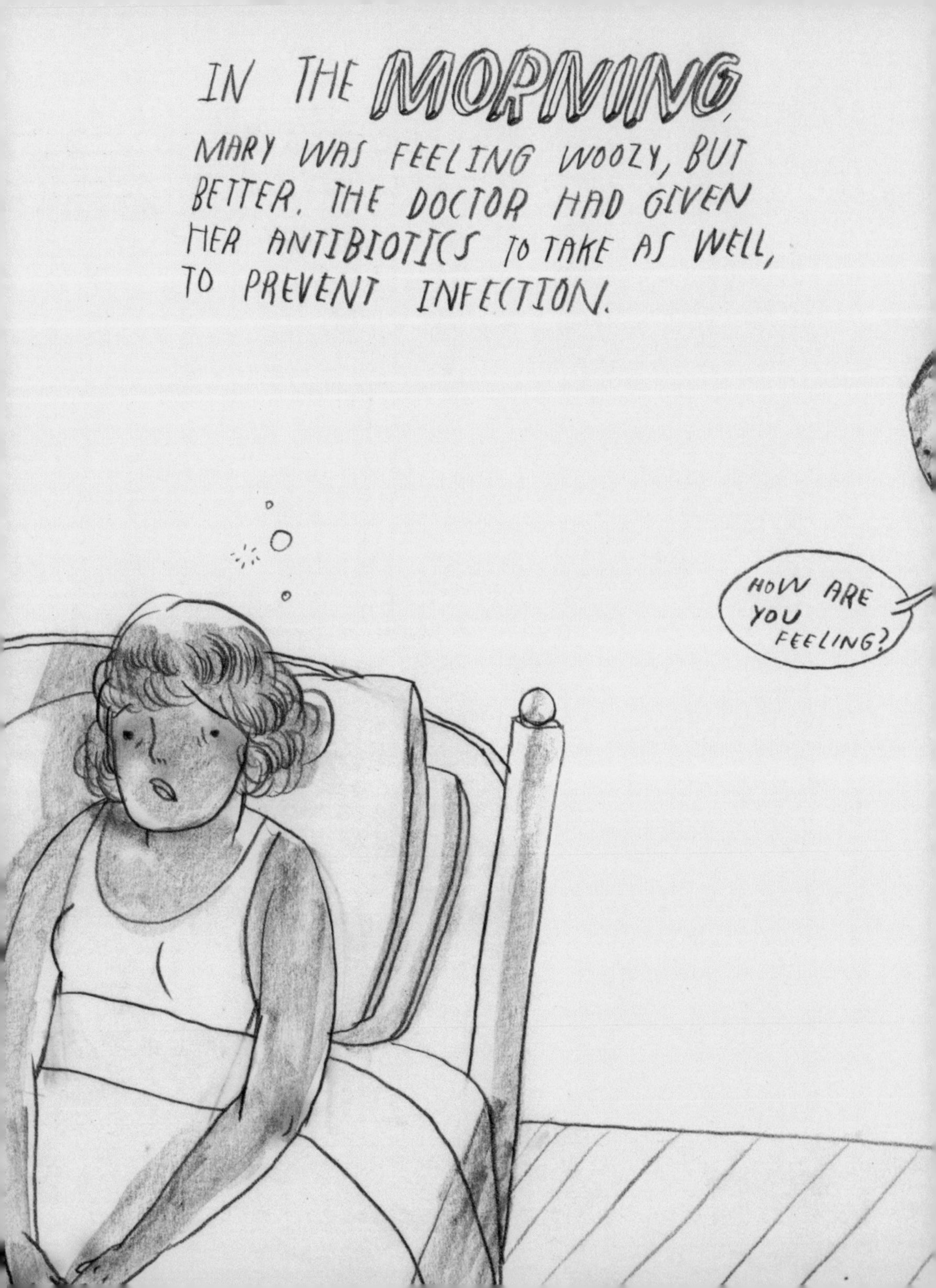
IN THE MORNING,
MARY WAS FEELING WOOZY, BUT BETTER. THE DOCTOR HAD GIVEN HER ANTIBIOTICS TO TAKE AS WELL, TO PREVENT INFECTION.
HOW ARE YOU FEELING?

OVER THE NEXT DAY (AND DAYS), MARY TOOK IT EASY. SHE DID NOT EXERCISE OR WALK FOR VERY LONG. SHE KEPT WEARING BIG PADS UNTIL THE BLEEDING FELT MORE LIKE A LIGHT PERIOD. LIKE LISA, SHE WAS NOT TO USE TAMPONS OR HAVE SEX FOR A WHILE.

MARY HAD A FOLLOW-UP CHECKUP WITH THE SAME DOCTOR A WEEK LATER. THIS IS A VERY IMPORTANT VISIT TO HAVE WHEN YOU HAVE A MEDICAL ABORTION AT HOME. THE DOCTOR NEEDS TO SEE IF THE PROCEDURE WAS SUCCESSFUL (COMPLETE), AND TO MAKE SURE YOU ARE FEELING HEALTHY.

...AND YOU DON'T FEEL ANY MORE ABDOMINAL PAIN..?
NO
CRAMPS?
NOPE
NAUSEA?
NO

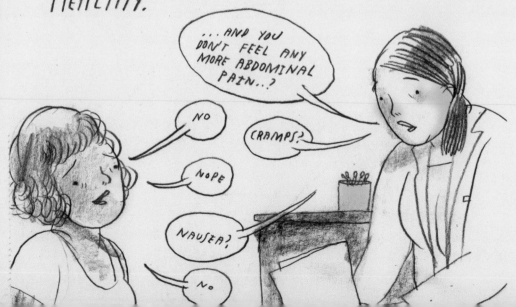

SHE WALKED HOME FROM THE OFFICE. SHE WANTED TO BE BY HERSELF AND THINK ABOUT EVERYTHING THAT HER BODY HAD BEEN THROUGH, AND WHAT IT ALL MEANT TO HER...

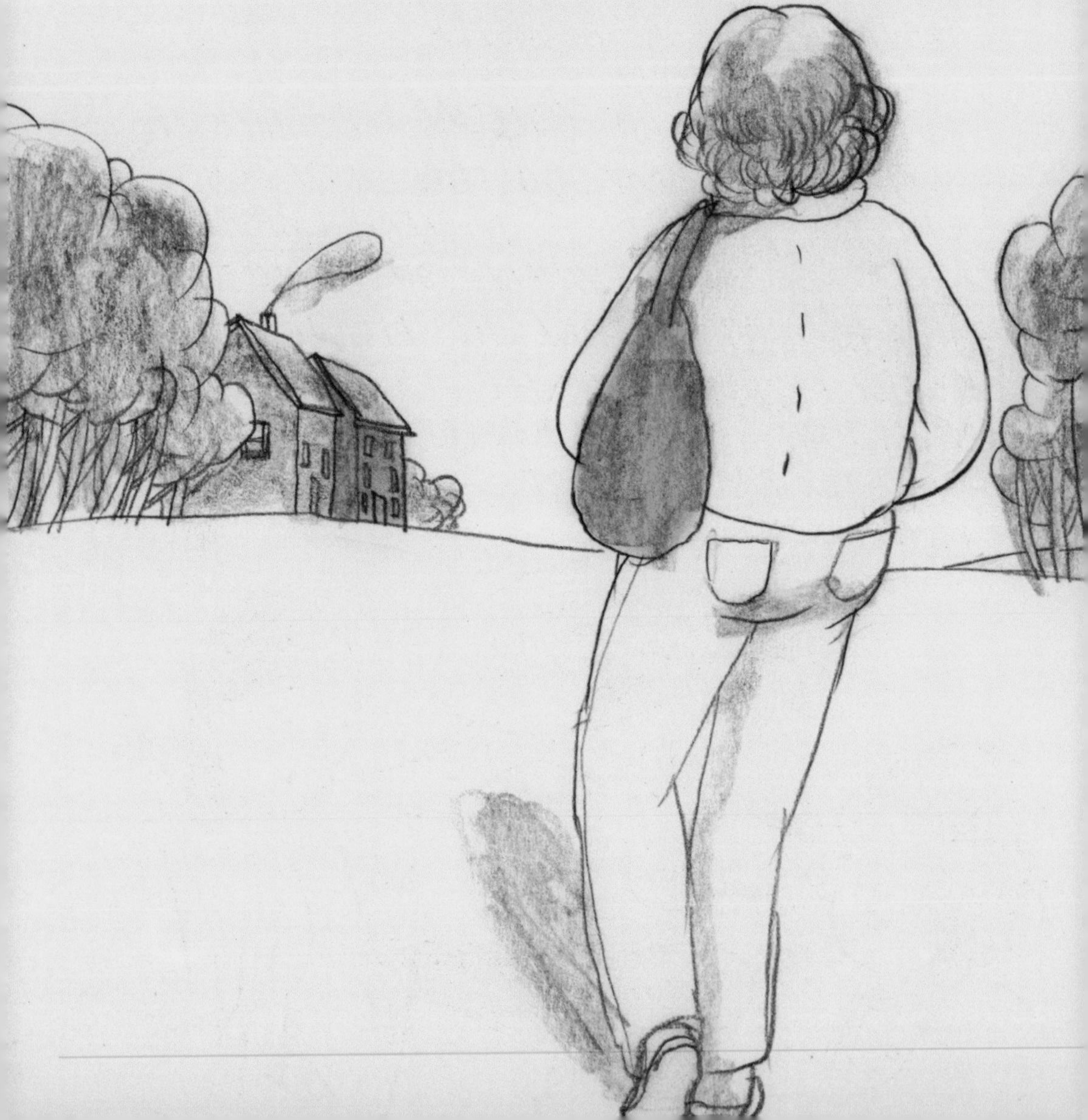

...BECAUSE SOMETIMES THAT
IS THE PART THAT TAKES US
THE LONGEST TO FIGURE OUT.

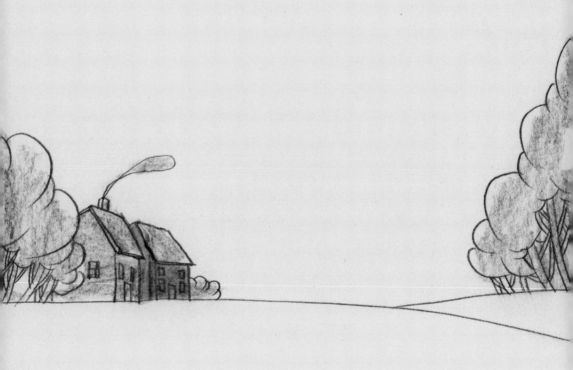

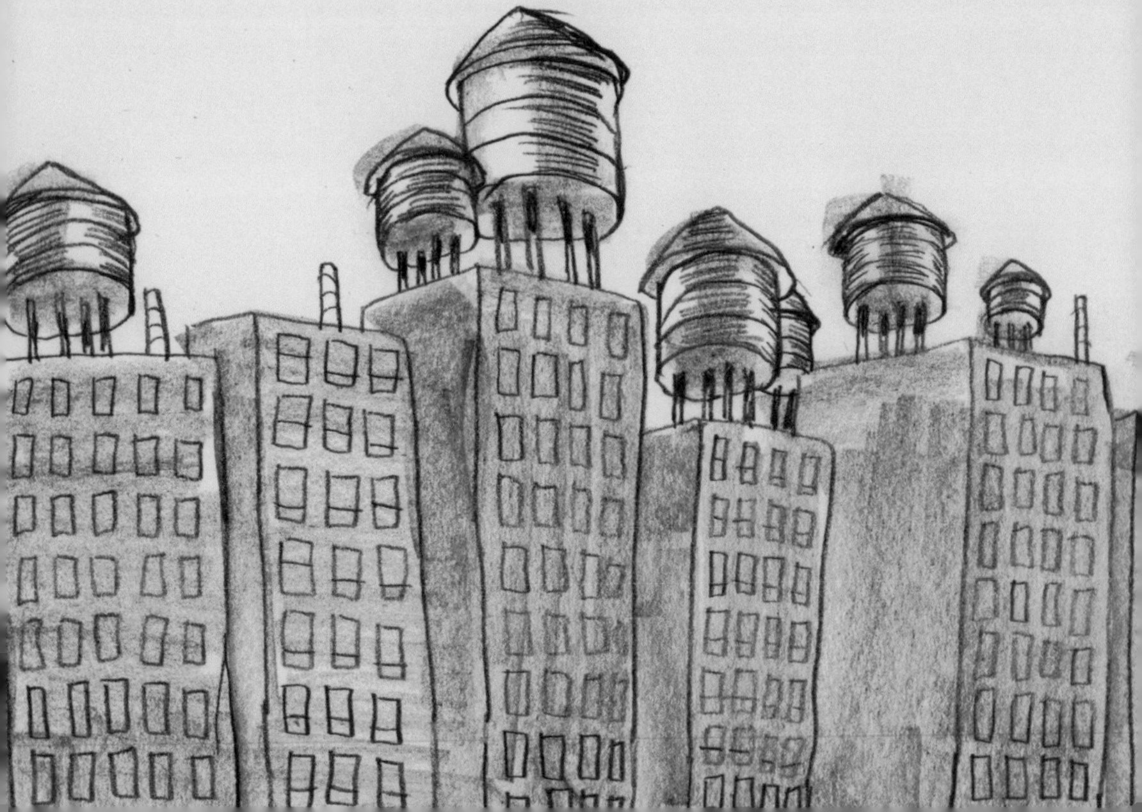

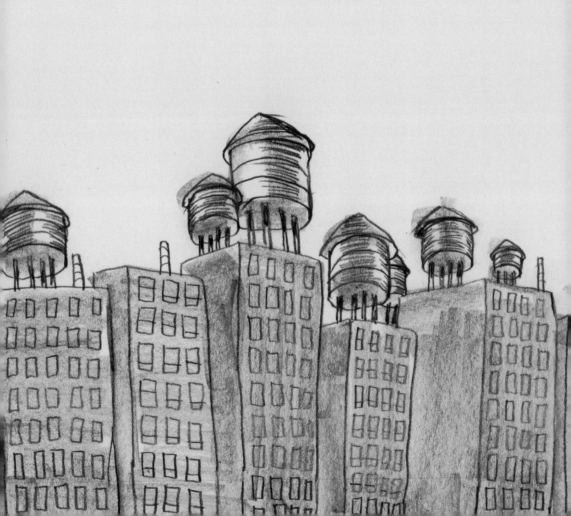

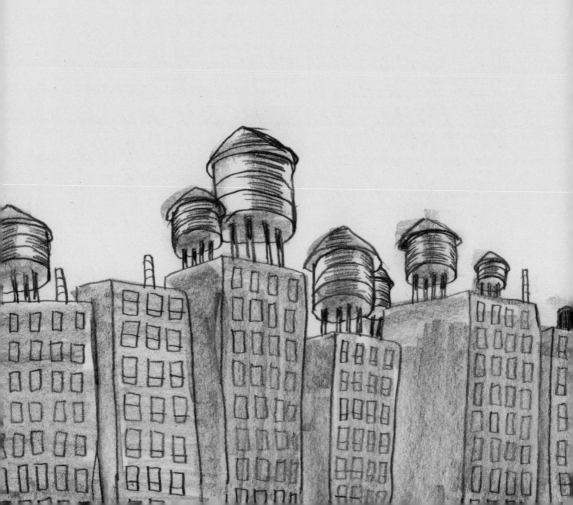

THANK YOU:

MOM, DAD, NINA, MIKE, THEO,
JESSIE, RACHIE, JOSH, ELSA, DIA, ANDREINA,
ALL HAYESES, BUBBA, MICHAEL LEVITON,
KYP MALONE, MYISHA, MARY ELLEN, ERIC &
GARY & EVERYONE AT FANTAGRAPHICS, BEN
RODGERS, ROB BRYN, MATT LITTLEJOHN, PARSONS,
ANDY KEHOE, AJ FOSIK, GARY BASEMAN,
JAY LEVINE, BRAD BANKS, BEN SHAPIRO,
SEAN WALSH, HEAVY DUTY, AMY SATHER,
PETERS DAY, DEVERY DOLEMAN, STEVEN
GUARNACCIA, SHARON VAN ETTEN, HEATHER
BRODERICK, AND PLANNED PARENTHOOD.

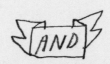

SPECIAL THANKS TO:
DEBORAH OYER AND
HEATHER CORINNA

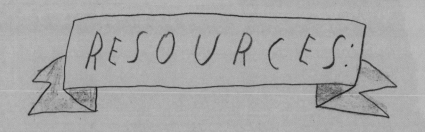

RESOURCES:

NATIONAL ABORTION FEDERATION:

WWW. PRO CHOICE. ORG

PLANNED PARENTHOOD:

WWW. PLANNEDPARENTHOOD. ORG

A YOUNG MAN'S GUIDE TO SEXUAL HEALTH:

WWW. PPFASTORE. ORG

BIRTH CONTROL/GENERAL:

WWW. WOMENSHEALTH. GOV

OTHER OPTIONS:

WWW. ADOPTION. COM

WHY THIS BOOK?

THERE ARE SEVERAL REASONS WHY I CHOSE TO WRITE THIS BOOK, AND THEN SHARE IT.

THE SUBJECT OF ABORTION IS A TRICKY ONE: SO MUCH (UNDERSTANDABLE) FOCUS IS GIVEN TO RIGHT/WRONG, SHOULD/SHOULDN'T, PRO/CON, CHOICE/NO CHOICE, ETC... THE POLITICAL DISCOURSE BEGINS ALMOST IMMEDIATELY AT THE DECISION WHETHER OR NOT TO ABORT, AND THEN OFTEN FLINGS ITSELF WILDLY TO THE "END" OF THE PROCESS. YOU DID IT: DID YOU DO THE RIGHT THING? ARE YOU CONFLICTED? WHAT DO YOU CALL YOURSELF, PRO-CHOICE OR PRO-LIFE? DO YOU HAVE REGRET, EITHER WAY? WHAT DOES IT MEAN TO REGRET HAVING AN ABORTION? WHAT DOES IT MEAN TO REGRET NOT HAVING AN ABORTION? THE SUBJECT IS LADEN WITH HEAVY, SOMETIMES UNANSWERABLE IDEAS AND QUESTIONS; BOTH HAPPY AND SAD, EMPOWERING AND SCARY.

AS FAR AS I UNDERSTAND IT:
A HUGE PART OF BEING ABLE
TO DECIDE FOR ONESELF WHETHER OR
NOT TO HAVE AN ABORTION IS THE
FREEDOM TO DEAL WITH SOME OF
THESE QUESTIONS AT YOUR OWN
PACE, IN YOUR OWN WAY, AT YOUR
OWN TIME.

BUT WHAT ABOUT THE
ACT "IN-BETWEEN" THE MEANING
AND THE POLITICS AND THE
ARGUMENTS? WHAT IS IT LIKE TO
GO THROUGH SOMETHING SO PHYSICAL
(YET SO EMOTIONALLY CHARGED),
SOMETHING SO PERSONAL, YET SOME-
THING SO UNIVERSAL...? A PROCEDURE
THAT SO MANY WOMEN GO THROUGH
CAN ALSO SEEM LIKE YOU ARE
VERY ALONE. PART OF MY INTENTION IS
TO MAKE SUCH A THING SEEM LESS
LONELY, IF I CAN.

AS THE AUTHOR, I'M NOT TRYING
TO OFFER MY OWN POLITICAL AGENDA
ONE WAY OR THE OTHER ABOUT
THE SUBJECT OF ABORTION, LIKE
YOU, I HAVE MY OWN THOUGHTS

AND FEELINGS SURROUNDING THE ISSUE. BUT ALSO LIKE YOU: THEY ARE PERSONAL, AND I WOULD NOT PRESUME TO SUGGEST YOU ADOPT MINE. WHAT I DO WANT IS TO SHOW MY OWN VISUAL INSIGHT INTO THE PHYSICAL PROCESS THAT WE DON'T ALWAYS GET TO SEE. MY GOAL IS TO SHOW, AND POSSIBLY, MAYBE COMFORT IN SOME WAY DURING AN EMOTIONAL PROCEDURE. I DO NOT TAKE THIS SUBJECT LIGHTLY. BUT I DO WANT GIRLS TO BE HEALTHY, HAPPY, MAKE GOOD CHOICES FOR THEMSELVES... AND ALL I HAVE IS A PENCIL.

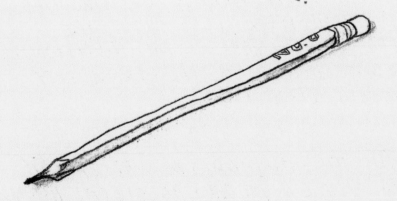

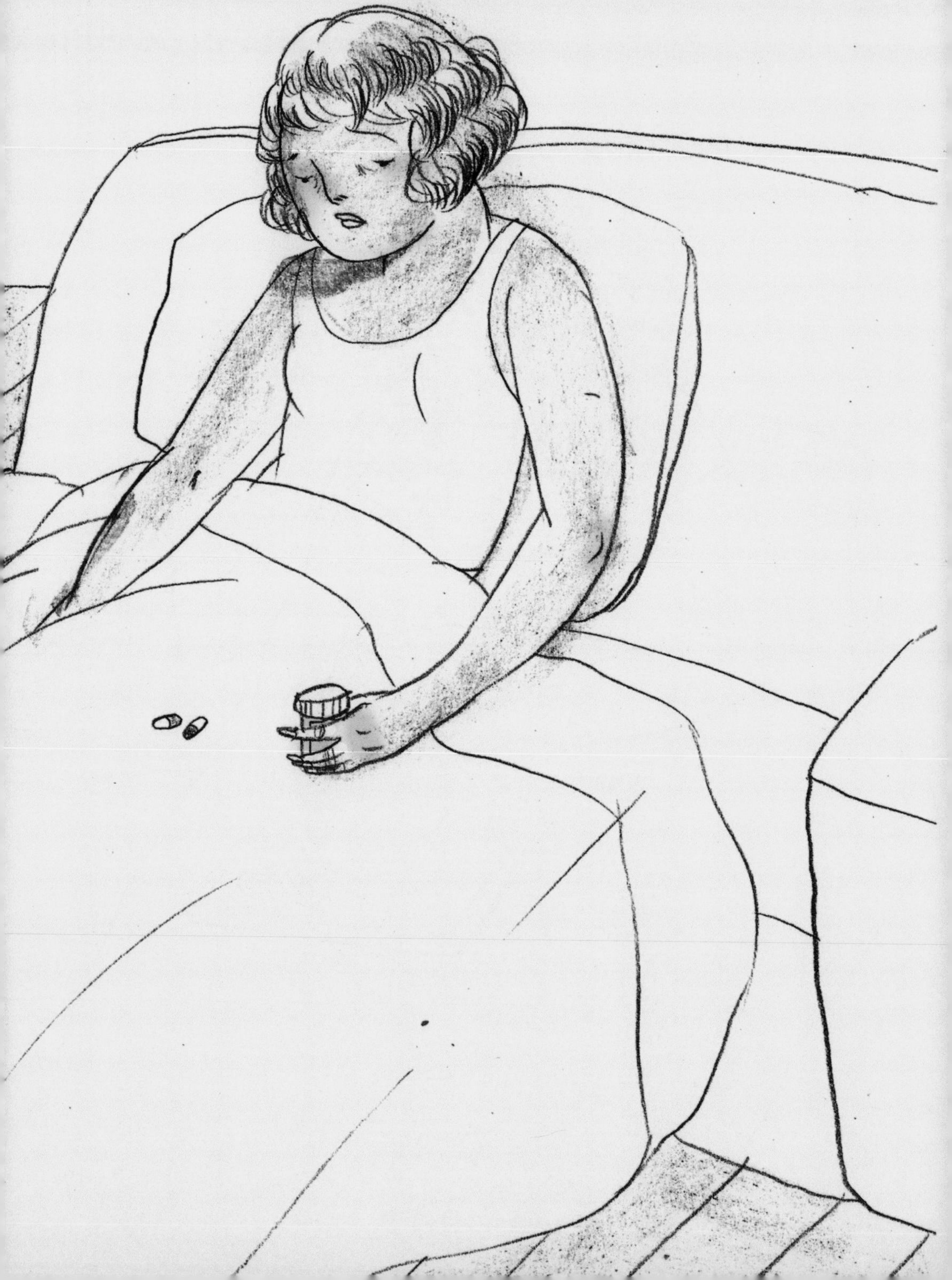

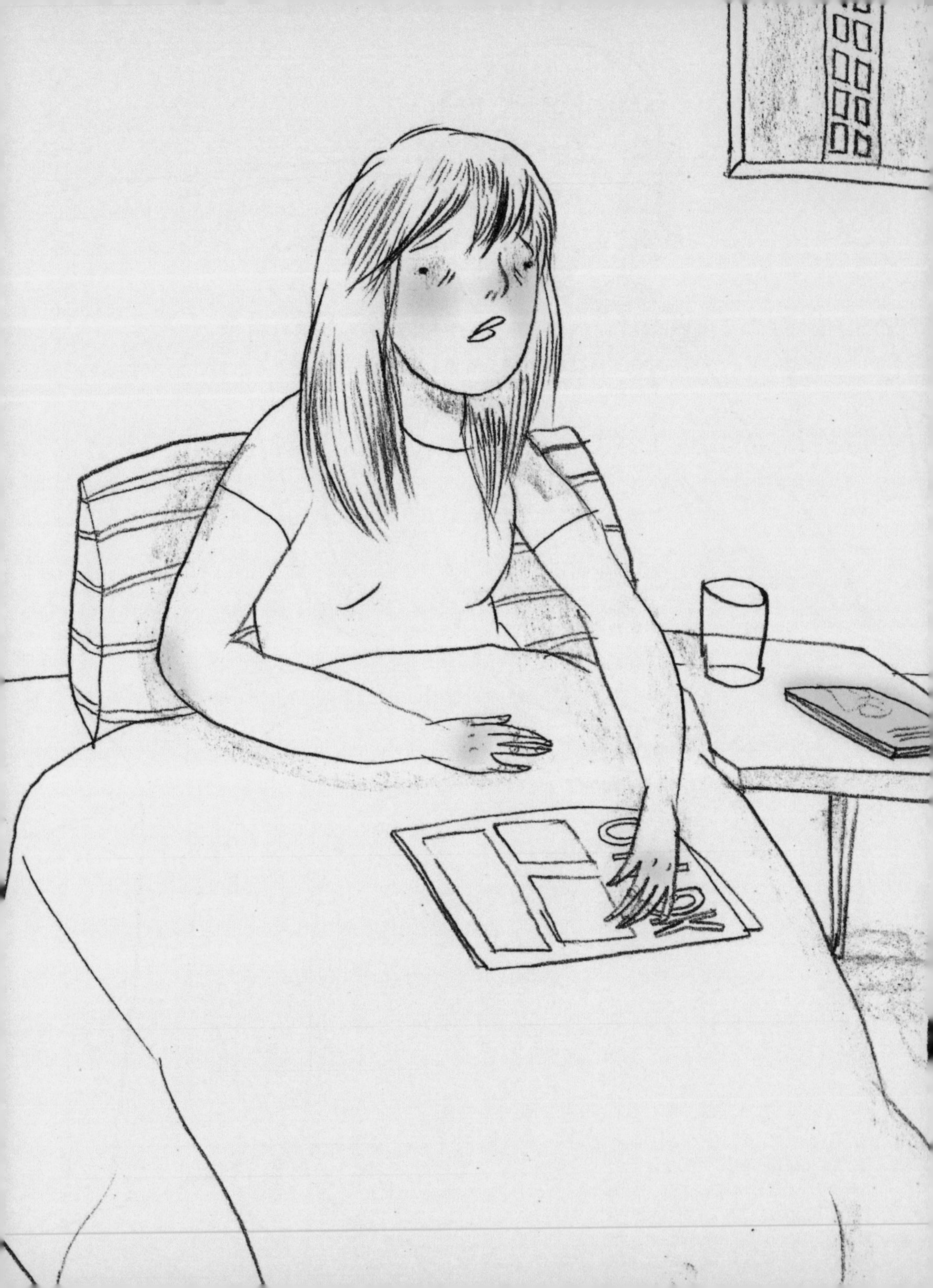

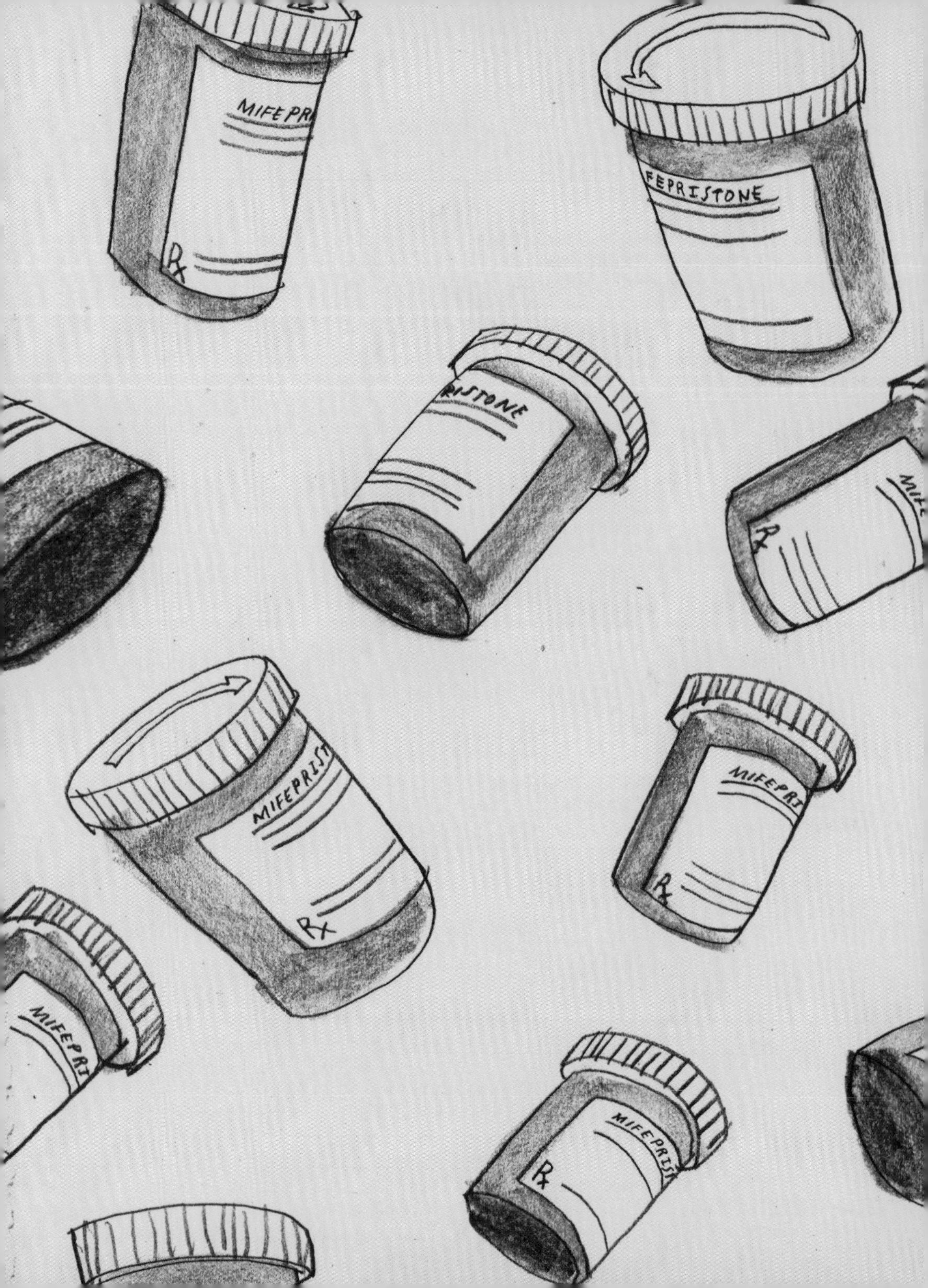
MIFEPRI
Rx
FEPRISTONE
RISTONE
Rx
MIFEPRIST
Rx
MIFEPRI
Rx
MIFEPRI
MIFEPRIST
Rx